INSTANT POT

VEGETARIAN RECIPES COOKBOOK

Unleash the complete Plant-Powered Kitchen: The Beginner's Guide to Instant Pot Vegetarian Cooking ~ Quick, Easy & Delicious Recipes for Busy People

DR JANE T. RYAN

INTRODUCTION

Greetings from the pleasant world of the Instant Pot Vegetarian Recipes Cookbook, a culinary adventure that honours flavour harmony, ease of preparation, and the pleasure of indulging. wholesome vegetarian meals with the convenience of your Instant Pot.

Embark on a gastronomic adventure with this carefully curated collection, where each recipe is a testament to the versatility and efficiency of the Instant Pot. Whether you're a seasoned chef or a kitchen novice, our cookbook is your go-to companion for crafting delicious vegetarian dishes that are not only nutritious but also bursting with taste.

As you flip through the pages, you'll discover a treasure trove of plant-based recipes that cater to diverse palates. From mouthwatering soups and stews to exotic one-pot wonders, each recipe is designed to bring out the best in your Instant Pot, making cooking a seamless and enjoyable experience.

What sets this cookbook apart is its emphasis on ingredients that are not only flavorful but also readily available. We believe in the power of accessible, wholesome ingredients to create extraordinary meals. Whether you're craving a quick weeknight dinner or planning a feast for family and friends, our cookbook has you covered.

To enhance your cooking experience, we've included helpful tips, cooking techniques, and stunning visuals that showcase the vibrant colors and textures of each dish. The artful presentation of recipes invites you to embark on a culinary journey that not only nourishes your body but also tantalizes your taste buds.

So, gather your ingredients, dust off your Instant Pot, and join us in creating a symphony of vegetarian flavors that will redefine your perception of home-cooked meals. The Instant Pot Vegetarian Recipes Cookbook is not just a collection of recipes; it's an invitation to elevate your culinary prowess and savor the joy of creating delicious, wholesome meals effortlessly. Happy cooking!"

OVERVIEW OF INSTANT POT COOKING

"In the realm of culinary innovation, the Instant Pot stands as a revolutionary kitchen companion, transforming the landscape of home cooking. As we delve into the captivating world of the Instant Pot Vegetarian Recipes Cookbook, let's explore the overarching principles that make Instant Pot cooking a game-changer.

Efficiency and Speed:

Instant Pot's claim to fame lies in its ability to drastically cut down cooking times. The ingenious combination of pressure cooking and advanced technology ensures that once-time-consuming recipes are now achievable in a fraction of the time. This efficiency becomes a cornerstone for busy individuals seeking a balance between a hectic lifestyle and nourishing, home-cooked meals.

Versatility in Vegetarian Delights:

Vegetarian cooking, often unfairly underrated, takes center stage in this cookbook. The Instant Pot proves to be an ideal vessel for enhancing the natural flavors of plant-based ingredients. From hearty lentil soups to succulent vegetable curries, the cookbook showcases a plethora of recipes that elevate vegetarian cuisine to new heights, debunking any notion of monotony in meatless meals.

Nutrient Retention:

Instant Pot's sealed cooking environment preserves nutrients that might be lost through traditional cooking methods. The controlled pressure and temperature ensure that vitamins and minerals remain locked into your dishes, promoting a healthier and more nourishing dining experience.

One-Pot Wonder:

The Instant Pot's multifunctionality shines as it seamlessly transitions from sautéing to pressure cooking, all within the same pot. This not only minimizes the number of dishes to clean but also allows for complex layering of flavors in a single pot, creating a symphony of tastes that will leave your palate in awe.

Navigating the world of Instant Pot cooking is made easy with its user-friendly interface. The cookbook complements this by offering clear instructions, handy tips, and cooking techniques that empower both beginners and experienced cooks alike to make the most of their Instant Pot.

In essence, the Instant Pot Vegetarian Recipes Cookbook is not just a compilation of delightful recipes; it's an homage to the transformative power of Instant Pot cooking. As we embark on this culinary journey, let the Instant Pot be your trusted ally, turning ordinary ingredients into extraordinary, flavorful masterpieces. Get ready to elevate your vegetarian cooking experience to new heights, one delectable recipe at a time."

BENEFITS OF VEGETARIAN RECIPES

"Embracing a vegetarian lifestyle extends beyond personal dietary choices; it's a conscious decision with a multitude of benefits for both individuals and the planet. As we explore the advantages of incorporating vegetarian recipes into your culinary repertoire, the depth and breadth of these benefits become apparent.

1. Health and Wellness:

Vegetarian diets, when well-balanced, are associated with a plethora of health benefits. They tend to be rich in essential vitamins, minerals, and antioxidants while being lower in saturated fats. Studies suggest that adopting a vegetarian lifestyle can contribute to improved heart health, better weight management, and a reduced risk of certain chronic diseases.

2. Nutrient Density:

Vegetarian recipes often feature a colorful array of fruits, vegetables, legumes, nuts, and seeds. This diversity ensures a broad spectrum of nutrients, including fiber, vitamins, and minerals. Consuming a nutrient-dense diet supports overall well-being and may contribute to increased energy levels.

3. Weight Management:

Vegetarian diets are naturally lower in calorie density and often higher in fiber, promoting satiety and aiding in weight management. Individuals following vegetarian recipes tend to have healthier body weight profiles and a lower risk of obesity.

4. Environmental Impact:

Choosing vegetarian recipes aligns with sustainability and environmental conservation. Deforestation, water pollution, and greenhouse gas emissions are all significantly impacted by animal husbandry. By opting for plant-based meals, individuals can reduce their carbon footprint and contribute to a more- eco-friendly food system.

5. Ethical Considerations:

For many, adopting a vegetarian lifestyle is rooted in ethical considerations. Choosing plant-based recipes aligns with a compassionate approach to animals, as it avoids the environmental and ethical concerns associated with industrialized animal farming.

6. Digestive Health:

Vegetarian diets, particularly those rich in fiber from fruits, vegetables, and whole grains, promote healthy digestion. Adequate fiber intake supports a balanced gut microbiome, reducing the risk of digestive issues and promoting overall gastrointestinal health.

7. Variety and Culinary Exploration:

Vegetarian cooking opens up a world of culinary exploration, encouraging creativity in the kitchen. With an abundance of plant-based ingredients, spices, and flavors, individuals can experiment with diverse recipes, expanding their palate and appreciation for a wide range of cuisines.

8. Long-Term Sustainability:

A vegetarian lifestyle is often seen as more sustainable for long-term health. It's a dietary choice that can be easily maintained throughout life, providing sustained health benefits and reducing the risk of certain age-related conditions.

The benefits of incorporating vegetarian recipes into your diet extend far beyond personal health. From environmental conservation to ethical considerations and culinary exploration, embracing a vegetarian lifestyle is a holistic choice that nurtures both individual well-being and the health of our planet."

1

Getting Started with Instant Pot

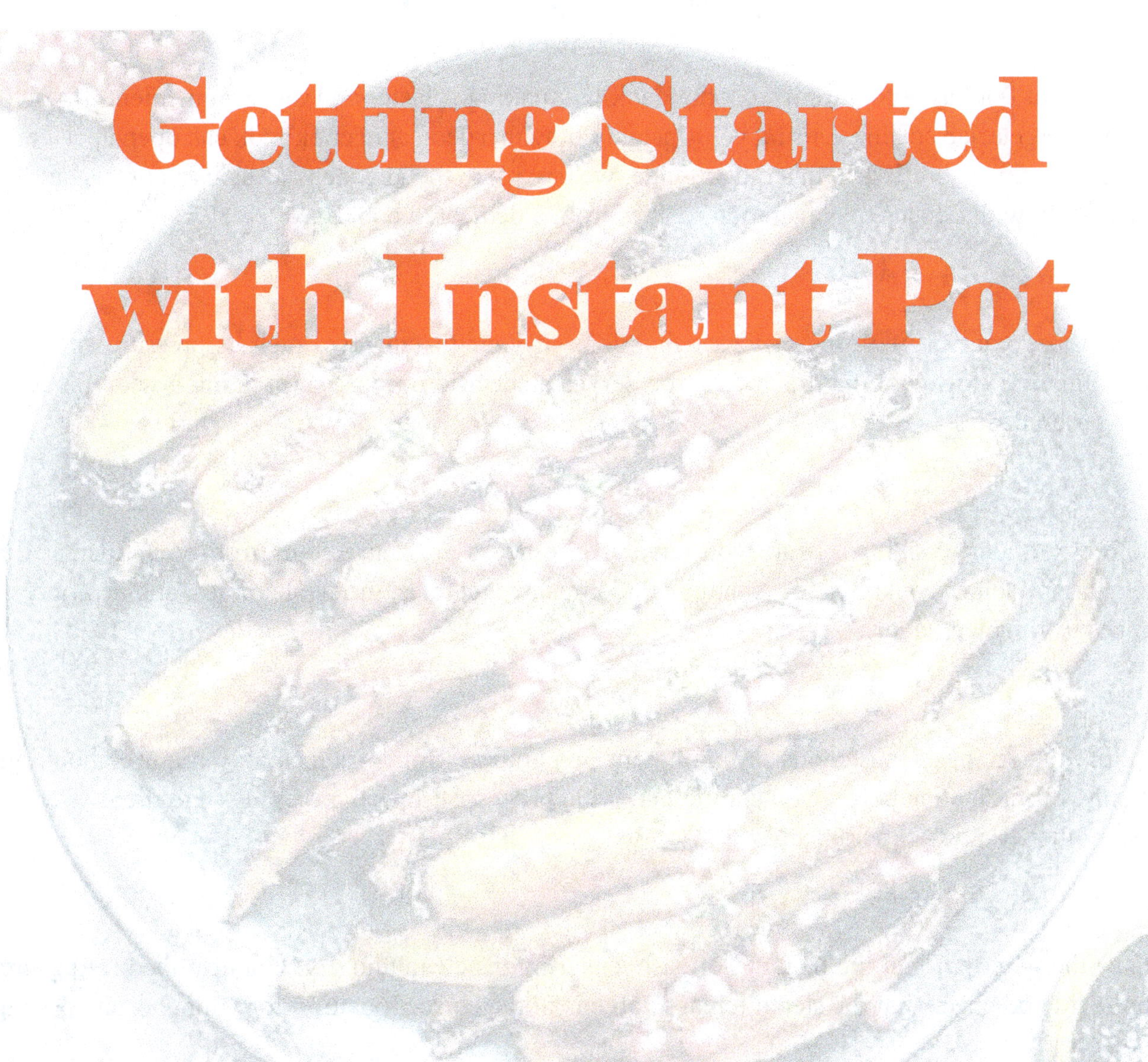

QUICK GUIDE TO USING THE INSTANT POT

The Instant Pot has revolutionized home cooking, making it faster and more convenient. If you're a fan of vegetarian cuisine, pairing your Instant Pot with a dedicated cookbook can open up a world of delicious possibilities. In this quick guide, we'll explore the key steps to using your Instant Pot effectively with a focus on vegetarian recipes from a dedicated cookbook.

Understanding Your Instant Pot:

Familiarize yourself with the different functions of your Instant Pot, such as pressure cooking, sautéing, and slow cooking. Each function serves a specific purpose in creating a wide range of vegetarian dishes.

Gathering Essential Ingredients:

Before you start cooking, ensure you have all the necessary ingredients from your Instant Pot vegetarian recipes cookbook. This may include fresh vegetables, grains, legumes, and a variety of spices to enhance flavor.

Prepping Ingredients:

Follow the recipe's instructions on ingredient preparation. Some recipes may require chopping, slicing, or marinating before you start the cooking process. Properly prepping ingredients ensures a smoother cooking experience.

Setting Up Your Instant Pot:

Place the inner pot into the Instant Pot base, ensuring it's clean and dry. Connect the sealing ring to the lid and check that the steam release valve is in the correct position for your chosen cooking method.

Programming Your Instant Pot:

Select the appropriate cooking function and time as per the recipe. Instant Pot vegetarian recipes often involve different cooking times for various ingredients, so pay attention to these details for optimal results.

Layer your ingredients in the Instant Pot according to the recipe instructions. Some recipes may require a specific order to ensure even cooking and flavor distribution.

Sealing and Cooking:

Close the Instant Pot lid, making sure it's properly sealed. Start the cooking process and let the Instant Pot work its magic. The pressure cooking feature is particularly efficient for reducing cooking time while preserving nutrients.

Natural or Quick Release:

After the cooking cycle completes, follow the recipe's recommendations for releasing pressure. Some recipes may suggest a natural release, while others benefit from a quick release to prevent overcooking.

Final Touches:

Once the pressure is released, open the Instant Pot carefully. Add any final ingredients or seasonings as directed by the recipe. Stir well and let the dish rest for a few minutes before serving.

Enjoying Your Meal:

Plate your Instant Pot vegetarian creation and savor the flavors. The Instant Pot's efficiency and versatility make it a valuable tool for exploring the diverse and tasty world of vegetarian cuisine.

By following these steps and embracing the recipes in your Instant Pot vegetarian cookbook, you'll unlock the full potential of this kitchen appliance, making meal preparation both convenient and enjoyable.

TIPS FOR SUCCESSFUL COOKING

Cooking with an Instant Pot can be a game-changer, especially when exploring the diverse realm of vegetarian recipes. To ensure success in your culinary adventures, consider these tips that specifically cater to the nuances of using an Instant Pot with a vegetarian recipes cookbook.

Read the Recipe Thoroughly:

Before diving into the cooking process, take a moment to read the recipe from start to finish. Understand the steps involved, required ingredients, and any specific Instant Pot functions needed. This ensures a smoother cooking experience.

Prep Ingredients in Advance:

Chop, slice, and measure all your ingredients before starting the cooking process. Instant Pot recipes often move quickly, and having everything ready in advance helps you stay organized and focused.

Use High-Quality Ingredients:

Invest in fresh, high-quality vegetables, grains, legumes, and spices. The Instant Pot has a way of intensifying flavors, so starting with premium ingredients will enhance the overall taste of your vegetarian dishes.

Layer Ingredients Thoughtfully:

Some recipes require layering ingredients to achieve even cooking. Follow the cookbook's instructions on how to arrange ingredients in the Instant Pot for optimal results. This is especially crucial for dishes with varying cook times.

Adjust Cooking Times and Temperatures:

Understand that cooking times may need adjustment based on factors like altitude, ingredient size, and personal preferences. Use the Instant Pot's customization options to fine-tune your cooking and achieve the desired texture and flavor.

Experiment with Seasonings:

Vegetarian dishes thrive on vibrant flavors. Try experimenting with different herbs, spices, and seasonings without hesitation. Taste as you go and adjust the seasoning levels to suit your palate.

The Instant Pot's sauté function is a versatile tool for enhancing flavors. Use it to brown vegetables, spices, or aromatics before pressure cooking. This extra step can elevate the overall taste and texture of your vegetarian creations.

Understand Pressure Release Methods:

Different recipes may call for natural or quick pressure release. Familiarize yourself with both methods and follow the cookbook's recommendations. Natural release is often suitable for dishes with delicate textures, while quick release may be ideal for others.

Invest in Accessories:

Consider purchasing Instant Pot accessories like steamer baskets, trivets, or silicone molds. These additions can expand your cooking possibilities and help you create a wider variety of vegetarian dishes with ease.

Document Your Successes:

Keep a cooking journal or notes on successful Instant Pot vegetarian recipes. Document any modifications you made, cooking times, and ingredient adjustments. This personalized record can serve as a valuable reference for future culinary endeavors.

Clean Your Instant Pot Regularly:

Maintain the integrity of your Instant Pot by cleaning it thoroughly after each use. Residue from previous meals can affect the flavors of new dishes, so keeping your Instant Pot in top condition is essential for successful cooking.

By incorporating these tips into your cooking routine, you'll be better equipped to unlock the full potential of your Instant Pot while exploring the delicious world of vegetarian recipes. Enjoy the process, embrace experimentation, and savor the delightful results of your culinary creations.

2

Breakfast Delights

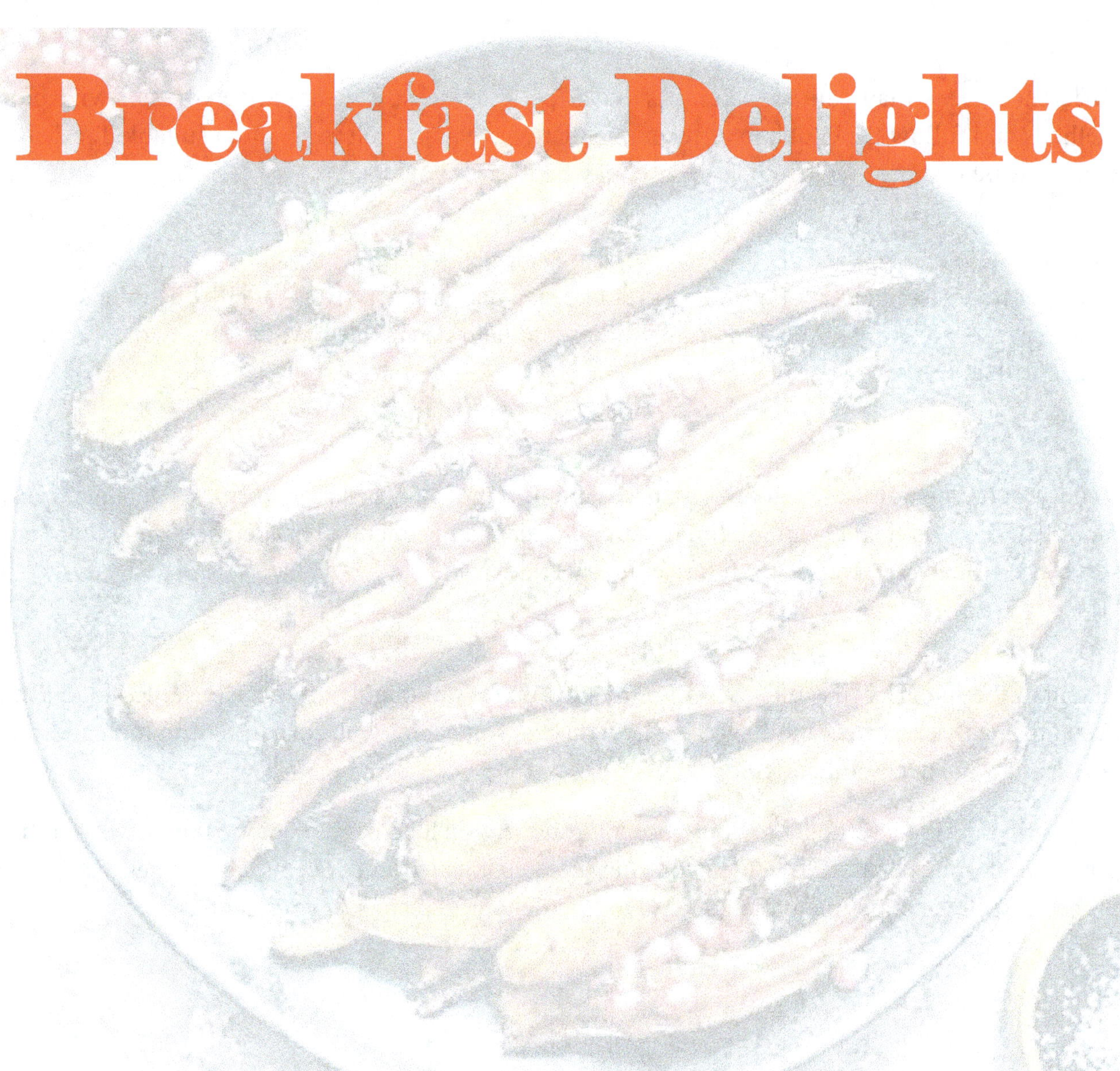

Quinoa Breakfast Bowl

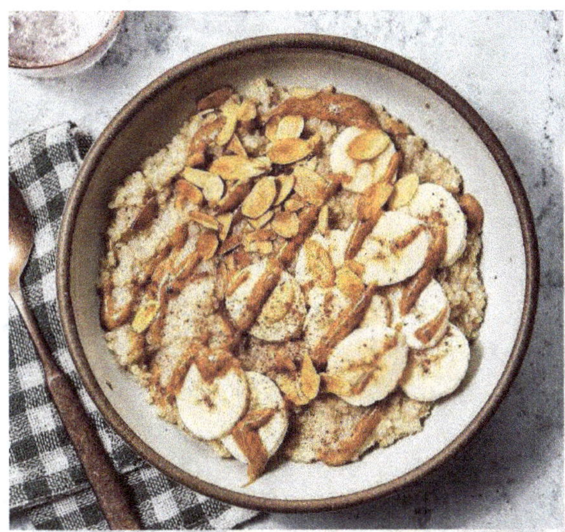

Ingredients:

- 1 cup quinoa
- 2 cups water
- 1 tablespoon olive oil
- 1 bell pepper, diced
- 1 cup cherry tomatoes, halved
- 1 cup spinach, chopped
- 4 eggs
- Salt and pepper to taste
  Optional toppings: avocado slices, feta cheese, salsa

Procedure:

- Rinse quinoa under cold water.
- In a saucepan, combine quinoa and water. After bringing to a boil, lower the heat to a simmer for fifteen minutes while covered.
- Heat the olive oil in a pan over medium heat.
- . Add diced bell pepper and sauté until softened.
- Add cherry tomatoes and spinach to the skillet, sauté until spinach wilts.
- In a separate pan, fry eggs to desired doneness.
- Combine cooked quinoa with the sautéed vegetables, season with salt and pepper.

- Divide the quinoa mixture into bowls, top each with a fried egg, and add optional toppings.

- Approximately 30 minutes.

Tips and Tricks:

- Customize toppings based on personal preference.
- Cook quinoa with vegetable or chicken broth for added flavor.

Nutritional Value per Serving:

- Calories: 400
- Protein: 18g
- Fiber: 8g
- Healthy fats: 12g
- Vitamins and minerals from vegetables.

Health Benefits:

- Quinoa provides complete protein and essential amino acids.
- Abundance of antioxidants from vegetables.
- Spinach is rich in iron and vitamins.

Packaging and Storing:

- Remaining food can be kept in the refrigerator for up to two days if it is sealed tightly.
- Warm up again on the burner or in the microwave.

Estimated Cost of Preparation:

- $10-$15 for four servings.

Precautions:

- Ensure quinoa is thoroughly rinsed to remove bitterness.
- Adjust salt levels based on personal dietary needs.

Post-Caution:

- Be mindful of allergens when choosing toppings.
- Incorporate variations to suit dietary preferences.

Instant Pot Oatmeal with Fruits

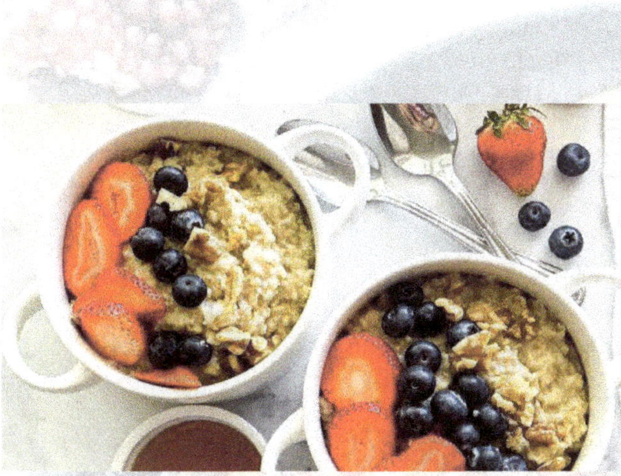

Ingredients:

- 1 cup steel-cut oats
- 3 cups water
- 1 cup milk (dairy or plant-based)
- 1 tablespoon maple syrup
- 1 teaspoon vanilla extract
- Pinch of salt
- Assorted fruits for topping (e.g., berries, banana slices, chopped apples)

Procedure:

- Combine steel-cut oats, water, milk, maple syrup, vanilla extract, and salt in the Instant Pot.
- Close the lid, set the Instant Pot to manual high pressure, and cook for 4 minutes.
- Allow natural pressure release for 10 minutes, then carefully release any remaining pressure.
- Stir the oatmeal, adjusting the consistency with additional milk if desired.
- Serve the oatmeal in bowls, topped with a variety of fresh fruits.

Time of Preparation:

- Approximately 20 minutes (including pressure build-up and release time).

- Use the Instant Pot's "Delay Start" feature for a ready-to-eat breakfast in the morning.
- Experiment with different fruit combinations for added variety.

Nutritional Value per Serving:

- Calories: 250
- Protein: 9g
- Fiber: 5g
- Healthy fats: 4g
- Rich in vitamins and minerals from fruits.

Health Benefits:

- Steel-cut oats provide sustained energy and are rich in fiber.
- Fruits contribute essential vitamins and antioxidants.
- Maple syrup adds natural sweetness without refined sugars.

Packaging and Storing:

- Remaining food can be kept in the refrigerator for up to three days if it is sealed tightly.
- Reheat in the microwave or on the stove, adding a splash of milk to restore creaminess.

Estimated Cost of Preparation:

- $5-$8 for four servings.

Precautions:

- Be cautious when releasing pressure from the Instant Pot to avoid burns.
- Adjust sweetness levels based on personal preference and dietary needs.

Post-Caution:

- Check the consistency after releasing pressure, adding more liquid if needed.
- Experiment with different fruit combinations for variety and added nutrients.

Eggless Frittata

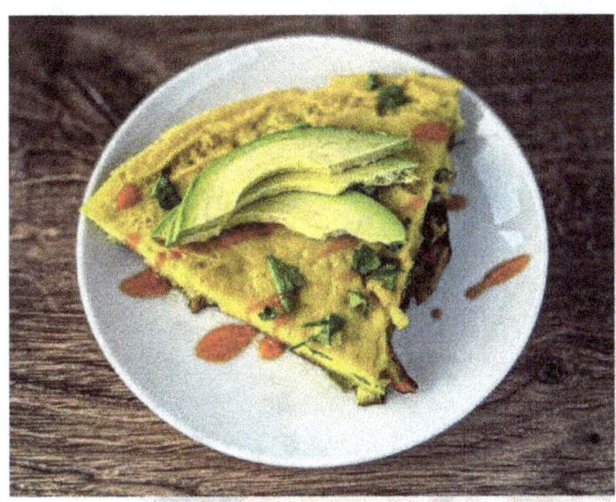

- 1 cup chickpea flour (besan)
- 1 1/2 cups water
- 1 tablespoon nutritional yeast
- 1 teaspoon baking powder
- 1/2 teaspoon turmeric powder
- 1/2 teaspoon black salt
- 1 tablespoon olive oil
- 1 onion, finely chopped
- 1 bell pepper, diced
- 1 cup cherry tomatoes, halved
- 1 cup spinach, chopped
- Salt and pepper to taste
- Optional: vegan cheese, herbs for garnish

Procedure:

- In a bowl, whisk together chickpea flour, water, nutritional yeast, baking powder, turmeric, and black salt until smooth.
- Heat the olive oil in an oven-safe skillet over medium heat.. Sauté onions until translucent.
- Add bell pepper, cherry tomatoes, and spinach to the skillet, sauté until vegetables are tender.
- Pour the chickpea flour mixture over the vegetables, ensuring an even distribution.
- Cook on the stovetop for 5 minutes, then transfer the skillet to a preheated oven (375°F or 190°C) and bake for 20-25 minutes until the frittata is set.
- Optional: sprinkle vegan cheese on top during the last 5 minutes of baking.

- Garnish with herbs, salt, and pepper to taste.

- Approximately 35-40 minutes (including baking time).

- Experiment with different vegetables for varied flavors and textures.
- Ensure the skillet is oven-safe before transferring to bake.

- Calories: 200
- Protein: 10g
- Fiber: 5g
- Healthy fats: 8g
- High in plant-based proteins and essential nutrients.

- Chickpea flour provides plant-based protein and fiber.
- Vegetables contribute vitamins, minerals, and antioxidants.

- Allow the frittata to cool before storing in airtight containers in the refrigerator for up to 3 days.
- Reheat in the oven or microwave.

- $8-$12 for four servings.

- Check the frittata's center with a toothpick to ensure it's fully cooked.
- Be cautious when handling the hot skillet.

- Adjust seasoning after baking if needed.
- Customize toppings or serve with a side salad for a complete meal.

3

Soups and Stews

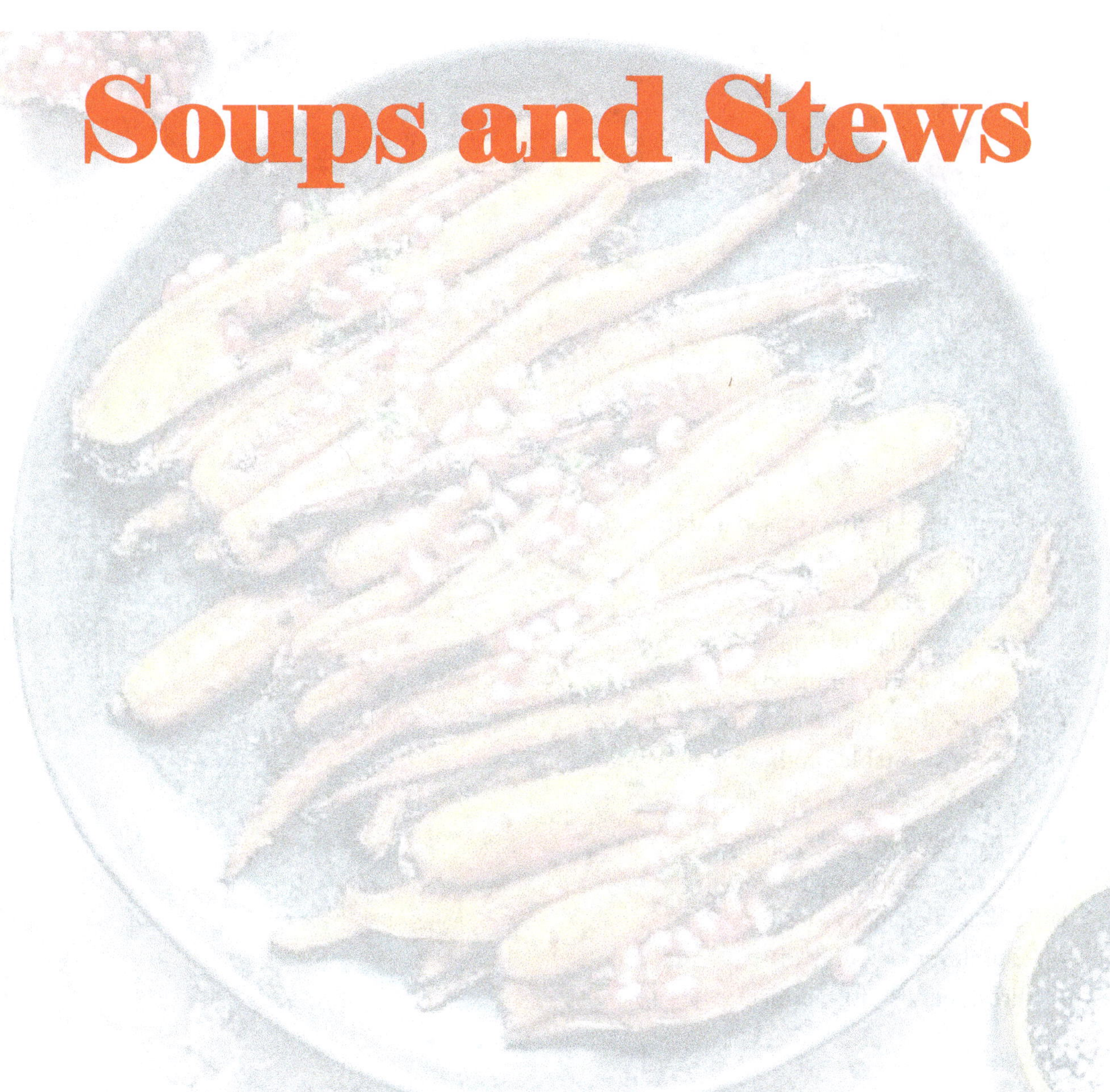

Lentil and Vegetable Soup

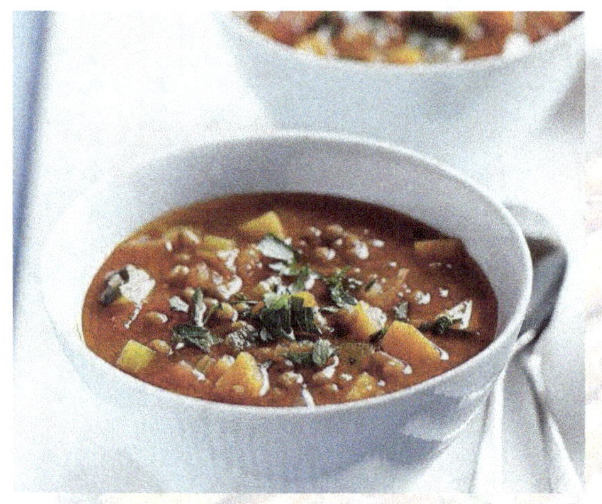

Ingredients:

- 1 cup dried lentils (rinsed and drained)
- 1 onion (chopped)
- 2 carrots (diced)
- 2 celery stalks (chopped)
- 3 cloves garlic (minced)
- 1 can (14 oz) diced tomatoes
- 6 cups vegetable broth
- 1 teaspoon ground cumin
- 1 teaspoon smoked paprika
- 1/2 teaspoon turmeric
- Salt and pepper to taste
- 2 tablespoons olive oil
- Fresh parsley for garnish

Procedure:

- In a large pot, heat olive oil over medium heat. Add onions, carrots, celery, and garlic. Sauté until vegetables are tender.
- Stir in lentils, diced tomatoes, vegetable broth, cumin, paprika, turmeric, salt, and pepper.
- Bring the soup to a boil, then reduce heat and simmer for 25-30 minutes or until lentils are cooked through.
- Adjust seasoning if necessary and serve hot, garnished with fresh parsley.

- Approximately 45 minutes.

- Soak lentils for a few hours before cooking to reduce cooking time.
- Customize with your favorite vegetables or add leafy greens for extra nutrition.
- Before serving, mix some of the soup for a creamier texture.

Nutritional Value per Serving (approx.):

- Calories: 250
- Protein: 13g
- Fiber: 10g
- Vitamin A: 80%
- Vitamin C: 25%
- Iron: 15%

Health Benefits:

- Rich in fiber, promoting digestive health.
- High protein content supports muscle development.
- Rich in antioxidants and vitamins for general health.

Packaging and Storing:

- Allow the soup to cool before transferring to airtight containers.
- Store in the refrigerator for up to 3-4 days or freeze for longer shelf life.

Estimated Cost of Preparation:

- $15-$20 (may vary based on location and ingredient quality).

Precautions:

- Check lentils for debris before cooking.
- Adjust salt levels according to personal dietary needs.

Post-Caution:

- Reheat thoroughly before consuming leftovers.
- Monitor portion sizes to align with dietary goals.

Tomato Basil Quinoa Soup

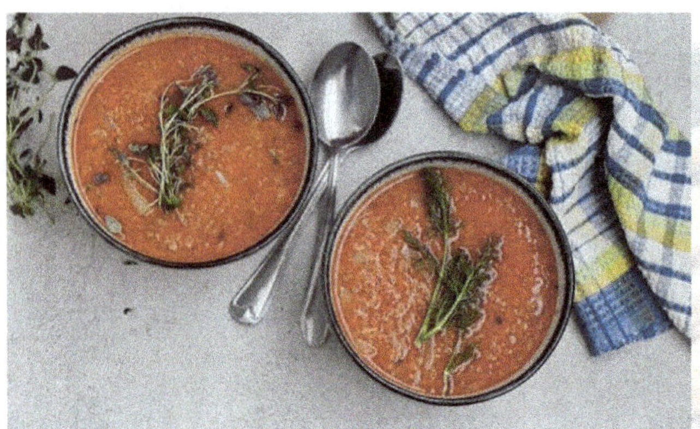

- 1 cup quinoa (rinsed)
- 1 onion (finely chopped)
- 2 carrots (diced)
- 3 cloves garlic (minced)
- 1 can (28 oz) crushed tomatoes
- 4 cups vegetable broth
- 1 teaspoon dried basil
- 1/2 teaspoon dried oregano
- Salt and pepper to taste
- 2 tablespoons olive oil
- Fresh basil leaves for garnish

Procedure:

- Warm up the olive oil in a big pot over medium heat. Add onions, carrots, and garlic. Sauté until onions are translucent.
- Add quinoa, crushed tomatoes, vegetable broth, dried basil, dried oregano, salt, and pepper.
- After bringing the soup to a boil, lower the heat, and simmer the quinoa for 15 to 20 minutes, or until it is tender.
- Adjust seasoning if necessary and serve hot, garnished with fresh basil.

Time of Preparation:

- Approximately 30 minutes.

- Toast quinoa in the pot before adding other ingredients for a nutty flavor.
- Customize by adding spinach or kale for additional nutrients.
- Use fire-roasted crushed tomatoes for a smoky twist.

Nutritional Value per Serving (approx.):

- Calories: 300
- Protein: 10g
- Fiber: 8g
- Vitamin C: 30%
- Iron: 20%
- Calcium: 8%

Health Benefits:

- Quinoa provides a complete protein source.
- Tomatoes are rich in antioxidants, promoting heart health.
- Basil adds anti-inflammatory properties.

Packaging and Storing:

- Allow the soup to cool before storing in airtight containers.
- Refrigerate for up to 4-5 days or freeze for longer storage.

Estimated Cost of Preparation:

- $12-$15 (may vary based on location and ingredient quality).

Precautions:

- Ensure quinoa is thoroughly rinsed to remove bitterness.
- Check canned tomatoes for added salt and sugar content.

Post-Caution:

- Be cautious with reheating to preserve the freshness of flavors.
- Monitor sodium intake, especially if using store-bought vegetable broth.

Chickpea and Spinach Stew

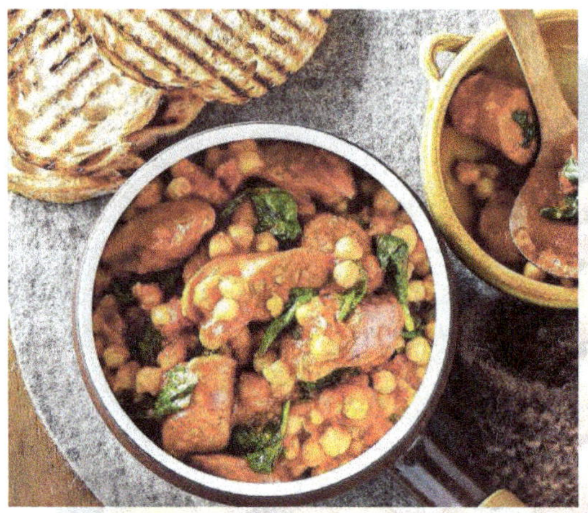

Ingredients:

- 2 cans (15 oz each) chickpeas (rinsed and drained)
- 1 onion (chopped)
- 3 cloves garlic (minced)
- 1 can (14 oz) diced tomatoes
- 1 cup vegetable broth
- 1 teaspoon ground cumin
- 1 teaspoon smoked paprika
- 1/2 teaspoon coriander
- Salt and pepper to taste
- 1 tablespoon olive oil
- 4 cups fresh spinach
- Lemon wedges for serving

Procedure:

- Warm up the olive oil in a big pot over medium heat. Add onions and garlic. Sauté until onions are softened.
- Add chickpeas, diced tomatoes, vegetable broth, cumin, smoked paprika, coriander, salt, and pepper.
- Bring the stew to a simmer and cook for 15-20 minutes.
- Stir in fresh spinach until wilted. Adjust seasoning if necessary.
- Serve hot, with a squeeze of lemon if desired.

- Approximately 30 minutes.

- Enhance flavor by adding a splash of balsamic vinegar.
- Try a variety of greens, such as Swiss chard or kale.
- For a thicker consistency, mash some chickpeas before adding spinach.

Nutritional Value per Serving (approx.):

- Calories: 280
- Protein: 12g
- Fiber: 10g
- Vitamin A: 70%
- Vitamin C: 25%
- Iron: 15%

Health Benefits:

- Chickpeas are a great source of plant-based protein and fiber.
- Spinach provides essential vitamins and minerals, promoting bone health.
- Rich in antioxidants, supporting overall immune function.

Packaging and Storing:

- Allow the stew to cool before storing in airtight containers.
- For extended shelf life, freeze or refrigerate for up to 3–4 days.

Estimated Cost of Preparation:

- $10-$12 (may vary based on location and ingredient quality).

Precautions:

- Check canned chickpeas for added salt and rinse thoroughly.
- Monitor sodium levels, especially if using store-bought vegetable broth.

Post-Caution:

- Reheat gently to avoid overcooking spinach.
- Be mindful of portion sizes for dietary considerations.

4

Appetizers and Snacks

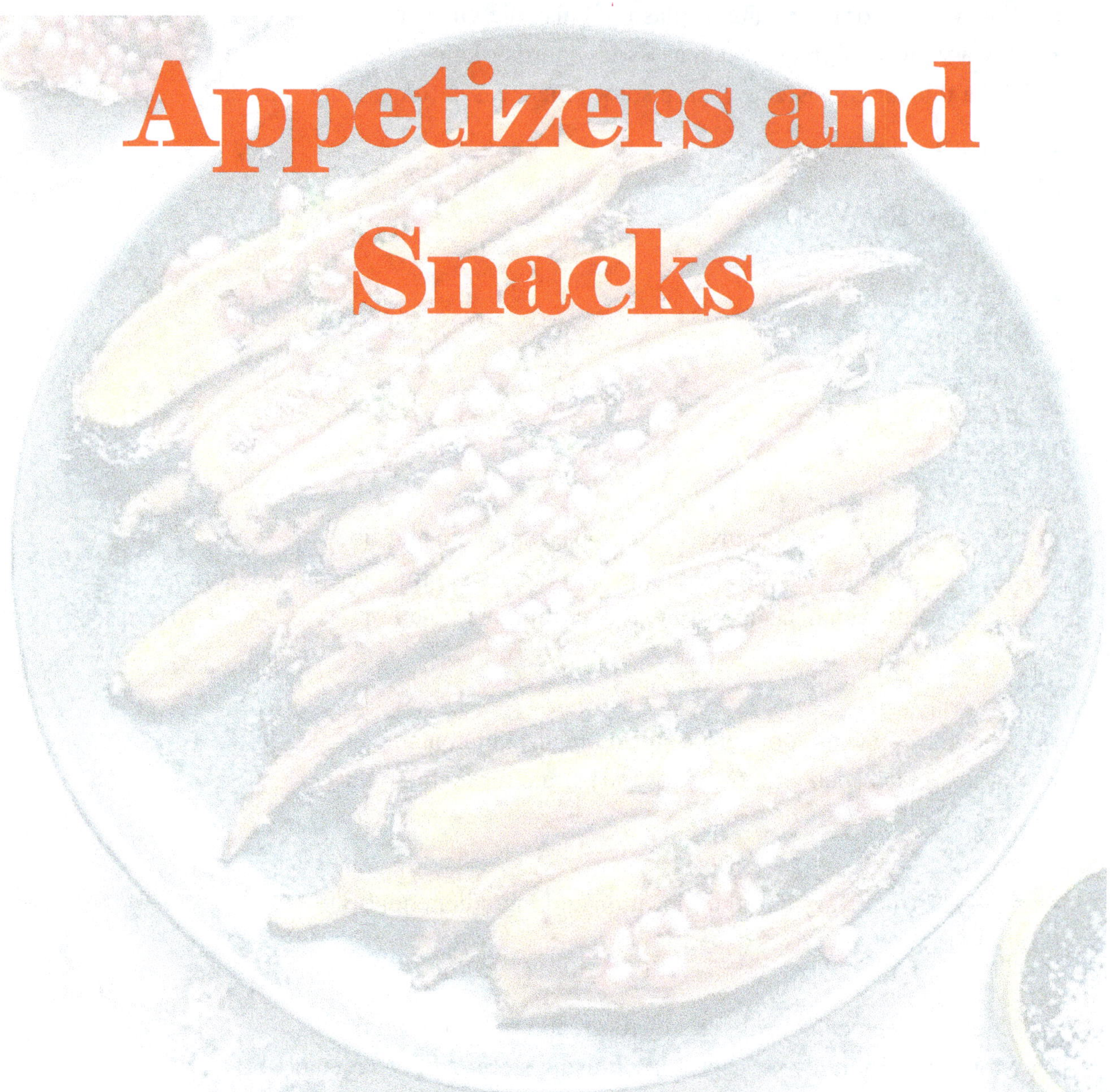

Stuffed Mushrooms

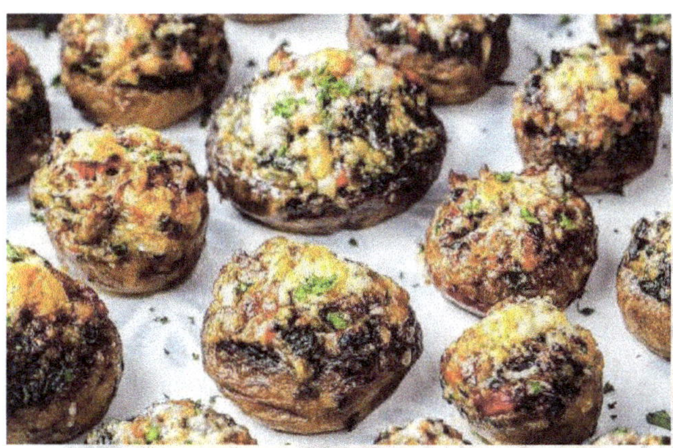

Ingredients:

- 24 large white mushrooms
- 1/2 cup breadcrumbs
- 1/4 cup grated Parmesan cheese
- 2 cloves garlic, minced
- 1/4 cup chopped fresh parsley
- 2 tablespoons olive oil
- Salt and pepper to taste
- 1/4 cup shredded mozzarella cheese

Procedure:

- Preparation: Preheat the oven to 375°F (190°C). Clean mushrooms and remove stems, creating a hollow space for stuffing.
- Filling Mixture: In a bowl, combine breadcrumbs, Parmesan cheese, minced garlic, chopped parsley, olive oil, salt, and pepper. Mix until well combined.
- Stuffing Mushrooms: Generously stuff each mushroom cap with the mixture, pressing down gently. The stuffed mushrooms should be put on a baking sheet.
- Baking: Bake for 18-20 minutes or until mushrooms are tender and the stuffing is golden brown. In the last few minutes of baking, sprinkle mozzarella cheese on top for a melty finish.
- Serving: Serve warm, and garnish with additional parsley if desired.

- Approximately 30 minutes.

- Choose mushrooms with firm caps to ensure they hold the stuffing well.
- Save the mushroom stems for other recipes like soups or sauces.
- Adjust the seasoning according to personal preference.

- Calories: ~70 kcal
- Protein: 4g
- Carbohydrates: 6g
- Fat: 4g
- Fiber: 1g

- Mushrooms are a good source of vitamins and minerals, including B-vitamins and selenium.
- Olive oil provides healthy monounsaturated fats.

- Remaining food can be kept in the refrigerator for up to two days if it is sealed tightly.
- Reheat in the oven for optimal crispness.

- $15 - $20, depending on the quality of ingredients and local prices.

- Ensure mushrooms are thoroughly cleaned to remove any debris.
- Be cautious while handling hot baking sheets and stuffed mushrooms.

- Be mindful of allergens like gluten and dairy in the ingredients.
- Practice safe food handling to prevent contamination.

Spinach Artichoke Dip

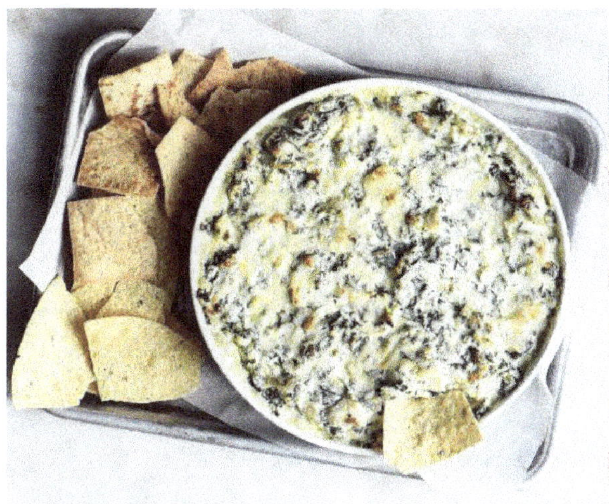

- 1 cup of thawed and drained frozen chopped spinach
- One can (14.2 oz) of drained and diced artichoke hearts
- 1/2 cup mayonnaise
- 1/2 cup sour cream
- 1 cup shredded mozzarella cheese
- 1 cup grated Parmesan cheese
- 1 teaspoon minced garlic
- 1/2 teaspoon onion powder
- 1/4 teaspoon black pepper
- 1/4 teaspoon salt
- 1/4 teaspoon red pepper flakes (optional)
- Tortilla chips or sliced baguette for serving

Procedure:

- Preparation: Preheat the oven to 375°F (190°C).
- Mixing Ingredients: In a large mixing bowl, combine drained spinach, chopped artichoke hearts, mayonnaise, sour cream, mozzarella cheese, Parmesan cheese, minced garlic, onion powder, black pepper, salt, and red pepper flakes if desired.
- Baking: Transfer the mixture into a baking dish and spread it evenly. Bake the dip for 25 to 30 minutes, or until the top is golden brown and the dip is hot and bubbling.

- To serve, take it out of the oven and allow it to cool down a little. Accompany with chopped baguette or tortilla chips.
- Advice and Techniques: To make a thicker dip, squeeze extra water out of the frozen spinach using a dish towel.
- Try a variety of cheeses to create a distinctive flavour profile.

Time of Preparation:

- Approximately 45 minutes.

Nutritional Value per Serving:

- Calories: ~120 kcal
- Protein: 4g
- Carbohydrates: 4g
- Fat: 10g
- Fiber: 1g

Health Benefits:

- Spinach is rich in iron, vitamins A and K.
- Artichoke hearts contain dietary fiber and antioxidants.

Packaging and Storing:

- Remaining food can be kept in the refrigerator for up to three days if it is sealed tightly.
- Reheat in the microwave or oven until well heated.

Estimated Cost of Preparation:

- $12 - $15, depending on ingredient quality and local prices.

Precautions:

- Ensure thorough draining of spinach and artichoke hearts to prevent excess moisture.
- Be cautious with hot baking dishes.

Post-Caution:

- Note any possible allergies in the ingredients.
- Practice moderation due to the calorie and fat content.

Sweet Potato Fries

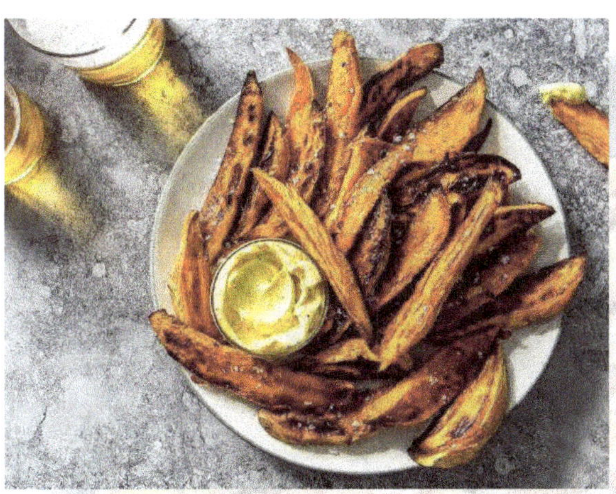

- 2 large sweet potatoes, peeled and cut into fries
- 2 tablespoons olive oil
- 1 teaspoon paprika
- 1 teaspoon garlic powder
- 1 teaspoon onion powder
- 1/2 teaspoon cayenne pepper (optional for heat)
- Salt and black pepper to taste

Procedure:

- Preparation: Preheat the oven to 425°F (220°C). Use parchment paper to line a baking sheet.
- Cutting Fries: Cut the peeled sweet potatoes into evenly sized fries, ensuring they are of similar thickness for even cooking.
- Seasoning: In a large bowl, toss the sweet potato fries with olive oil, paprika, garlic powder, onion powder, cayenne pepper (if using), salt, and black pepper. Ensure the fries are well-coated.
- Baking: Arrange the fries on the prepared baking sheet in a single layer, taking care not to pack them too tightly. Bake for 25 to 30 minutes, rotating them halfway through, or until they are crispy and golden.
- Serving: Remove from the oven and serve immediately. Enjoy with your favorite dipping sauce.

- Approximately 40 minutes.

Tips and Tricks:

- Soak the cut sweet potatoes in cold water for 30 minutes to remove excess starch, resulting in crispier fries.
- Use a parchment paper-lined baking sheet for easy cleanup.

Nutritional Value per Serving:

- Calories: ~150 kcal
- Carbohydrates: 26g
- Fat: 5g
- Fiber: 4g
- Protein: 2g

Health Benefits:

- Sweet potatoes are rich in vitamins A and C, fiber, and antioxidants.
- Olive oil provides heart-healthy monounsaturated fats.

Packaging and Storing:

- Allow fries to cool completely before storing in an airtight container in the refrigerator for up to 2 days.
- Reheat in the oven to maintain crispiness.

Estimated Cost of Preparation:

- $5 - $7, depending on ingredient quality and local prices.

Precautions:

- Watch the fries closely in the last few minutes to avoid burning.
- Be cautious when handling hot baking sheets.

Post-Caution:

- Note any possible allergies in the ingredients.
- Practice moderation due to the caloric content of the olive oil.

5
One-Pot Pastas

Creamy Garlic Alfredo Pasta

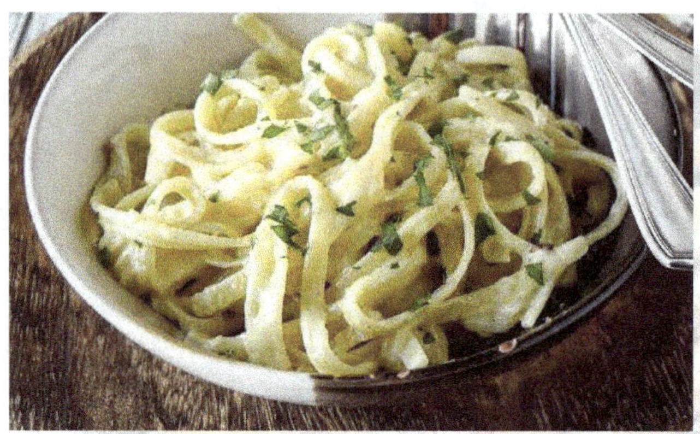

Ingredients:

- 8 oz fettuccine pasta
- 1/2 cup unsalted butter
- 4 cloves garlic, minced
- 2 cups heavy cream
- 1 cup grated Parmesan cheese
- Salt and black pepper to taste
- Fresh parsley for garnish

Procedure:

- Boil fettuccine pasta according to package instructions. Drain and set aside.
- Melt butter in a big skillet over a medium heat. When aromatic, add the minced garlic and sauté it.
- Add the heavy cream while continuously stirring. Heat to a low simmer.
- Add the Parmesan cheese gradually while whisking until smooth and creamy.
- To taste, add salt and black pepper for seasoning.
- Toss the cooked pasta into the sauce to ensure it is uniformly coated.
- Garnish with fresh parsley and serve hot.

Time of Preparation:

- Approximately 20-25 minutes.

- Use fresh Parmesan for a richer flavor.
- Adjust the consistency by adding more cream if needed.
- Be cautious with salt, as Parmesan is already salty.

Nutritional Value per Serving:

- Calories: 600 kcal
- Fat: 45g
- Carbohydrates: 35g
- Protein: 15g

Health Benefits:

- Good source of calcium and protein from Parmesan.
- Moderation is key due to the richness of the dish.

Packaging and Storing:

- For up to two days, store in the refrigerator in airtight containers.
- Reheat gently on the stove, adding a splash of cream to retain creaminess.

Estimated Cost of Preparation:

- Approximately $15 for four servings.

Precautions:

- Be mindful of butter and cream intake for those with dietary restrictions.
- Check for garlic allergies.

Post Caution:

- Moderate consumption due to high-calorie content.
- Consider lighter alternatives for regular consumption.

Ratatouille Pasta

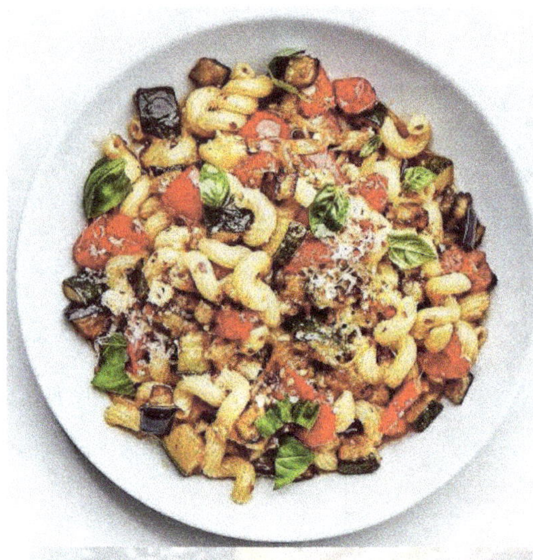

Ingredients:

- 8 oz penne pasta
- 1 medium eggplant, diced
- 1 medium zucchini, diced
- 1 bell pepper (any color), diced
- 1 large tomato, diced
- 1 onion, finely chopped
- 3 cloves garlic, minced
- 1/4 cup olive oil
- 1 tsp dried oregano
- 1 tsp dried basil
- Salt and black pepper to taste
- Grated Parmesan cheese for serving

Procedure:

- Cook penne pasta according to package instructions. Drain and set aside.
- Heat the olive oil in a big skillet over medium heat.. Add garlic and onion, sauté until softened.
- Add diced eggplant, zucchini, bell pepper, and tomatoes. Cook until vegetables are tender.
- Season with dried oregano, basil, salt, and black pepper. Stir well.

- Combine the cooked pasta with the ratatouille mixture, tossing to blend flavors.
- Serve hot, topped with grated Parmesan cheese.

Time of Preparation:

- Approximately 25-30 minutes.

Tips and Tricks:

- Cut vegetables uniformly for even cooking.
- Allow the veggies to caramelize for enhanced flavor.
- Adjust seasoning to personal preference.

Nutritional Value per Serving:

- Calories: 400 kcal
- Fat: 12g
- Carbohydrates: 65g
- Protein: 12g

Health Benefits:

- Rich in fiber, vitamins, and antioxidants from assorted vegetables.
- Low in saturated fats, suitable for heart health.

Packaging and Storing:

- Remaining food can be kept in the refrigerator for up to three days if it is sealed tightly.
- Reheat in a pan with a splash of water to maintain texture.

Estimated Cost of Preparation:

- Approximately $12 for four servings.

Precautions:

- Watch salt intake, especially if using Parmesan cheese.
- Adjust oil quantity for those watching caloric intake.

Post Caution:

- Incorporate as part of a balanced diet.
- Suitable for vegetarians.
- Indulge in this flavorful Ratatouille Pasta with these comprehensive guidelines!

Spinach and Tomato Linguine

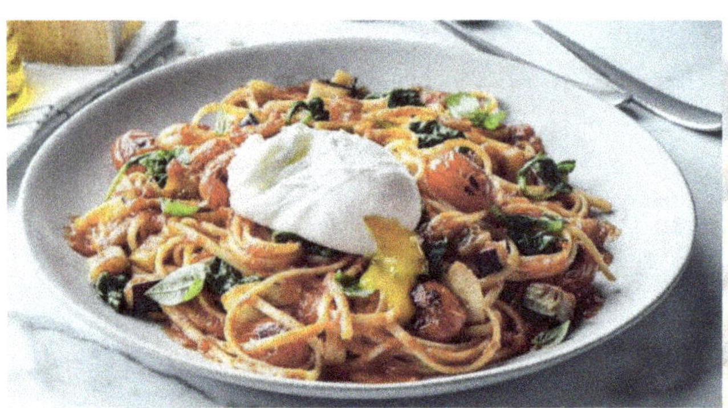

Ingredients:

- 8 oz linguine pasta
- 2 cups fresh spinach, chopped
- 1 cup cherry tomatoes, halved
- 3 cloves garlic, minced
- 1/4 cup olive oil
- 1/4 cup grated Parmesan cheese
- Red pepper flakes (optional)
- Salt and black pepper to taste
- Fresh basil for garnish

Procedure:

- Cook linguine pasta according to package instructions. Drain and set aside.
- Heat the olive oil in a big skillet over medium heat. When aromatic, add the minced garlic and sauté it.
- Add cherry tomatoes to the skillet, cooking until slightly softened.
- Toss in chopped spinach and cook until wilted.
- Combine cooked linguine with the tomato and spinach mixture, tossing well.
- If preferred, add red pepper flakes, black pepper, and salt for seasoning.
- Sprinkle grated Parmesan cheese on top and garnish with fresh basil.

Time of Preparation:

- Approximately 20-25 minutes.

- Use whole wheat linguine for added fiber.
- Adjust spice levels with red pepper flakes to taste.
- Fresh, ripe tomatoes enhance flavor.

Nutritional Value per Serving:

- Calories: 350 kcal
- Fat: 12g
- Carbohydrates: 45g
- Protein: 10g

Health Benefits:

- Rich in vitamins and antioxidants from spinach and tomatoes.
- Olive oil provides heart-healthy monounsaturated fats.

Packaging and Storing:

- For up to two days, keep in the refrigerator in an airtight container.
- Reheat with a splash of water on low heat on the stove.

.Estimated Cost of Preparation:

- Approximately $10 for four servings.

Precautions:

- Be mindful of salt if using Parmesan cheese.
- Check for spinach allergies.

Post Caution:

- Suitable for a light and nutritious meal.
- Great for incorporating leafy greens into the diet.

6

Rice and Grains

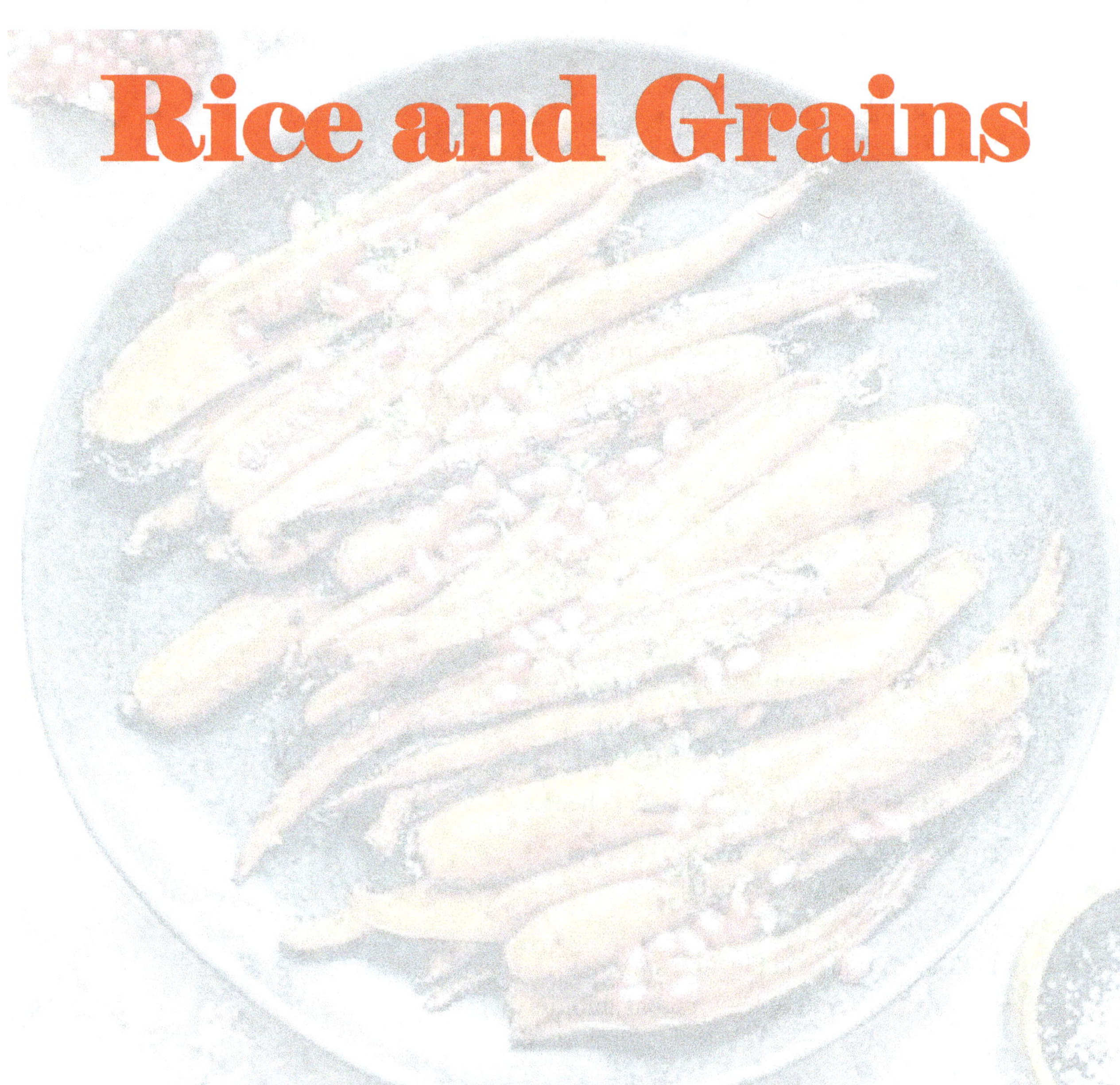

Vegetable Biryani

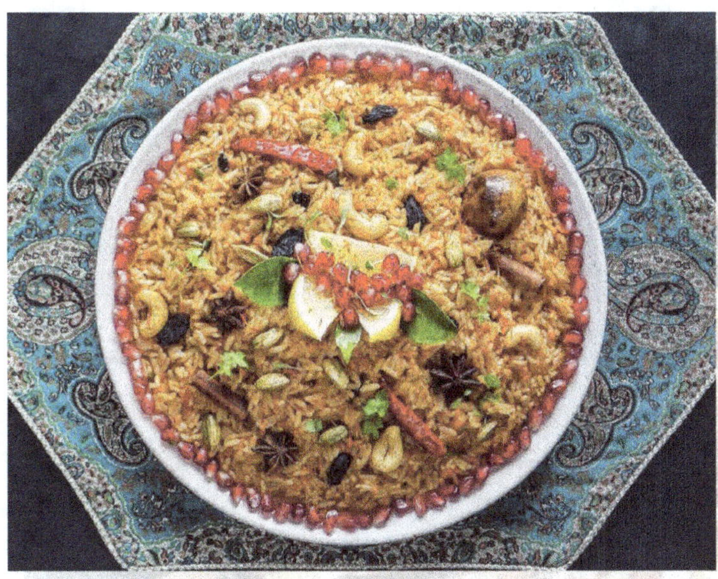

Ingredients:

- 2 cups basmati rice
- One cup of mixed veggies, such as potatoes, carrots, peas, and beans
- 1 large onion, thinly sliced
- 2 tomatoes, chopped
- 1/2 cup plain yogurt
- 1/4 cup chopped mint leaves
- 1/4 cup chopped coriander leaves
- 4 cups water
- 1/4 cup ghee or oil
- 1 tablespoon ginger-garlic paste
- 1 teaspoon cumin seeds
- 4-5 green cardamom pods
- 4-5 cloves
- 2-inch cinnamon stick
- 1 bay leaf
- 1/2 teaspoon turmeric powder
- 1 teaspoon red chili powder
- 1 teaspoon garam masala

- Salt to taste

Procedure:

- Till the water runs clear, rinse the basmati rice under cold water. After soaking in water for half an hour, strain the rice.
- In a large pot, heat ghee/oil, add cumin seeds, cardamom, cloves, cinnamon, and bay leaf. Sauté until aromatic.
- Add sliced onions and cook until golden brown. Add ginger-garlic paste, tomatoes, and cook until tomatoes are soft.
- Add mixed vegetables, turmeric powder, red chili powder, and salt. Cook for 5-7 minutes.
- Stir in yogurt, mint, and coriander leaves. Cook for an additional 2 minutes.
- Add soaked and drained rice to the pot. Mix gently to coat the rice with the spices.
- Pour water, bring to a boil, then reduce heat to low, cover, and simmer until rice is cooked and water is absorbed.
- Sprinkle garam masala, cover, and let it rest for 5 minutes. Fluff the rice with a fork.

Time of Preparation:

- Approximately 45-50 minutes.

Tips and Tricks:

- Use aged basmati rice for better texture.
- Adjust spice levels according to personal preference.
- Ensure vegetables are evenly chopped for uniform cooking.

Nutritional Value (Per Serving):

- Calories: ~350
- Protein: ~7g
- Carbohydrates: ~65g
- Fat: ~7g
- Fiber: ~5g

Health Benefits:

- Rich in vitamins and minerals from vegetables.
- Basmati rice provides a good source of energy.
- Yogurt contributes to gut health.

Packaging and Storing:

- Store in an airtight container in the refrigerator for up to 2-3 days.
- Freeze for longer shelf life; reheat in a pan or microwave.

Estimated Cost of Preparation:

- Depending on location and ingredient quality, approximately $15-20.

Precautions:

- Ensure vegetables are thoroughly washed.
- Adjust spice levels for dietary restrictions.
- Be cautious with hot utensils during the cooking process.

Post Caution:

- Allow biryani to cool before storing to prevent condensation.
- Reheat thoroughly before consumption.

Mexican Quinoa Bowl

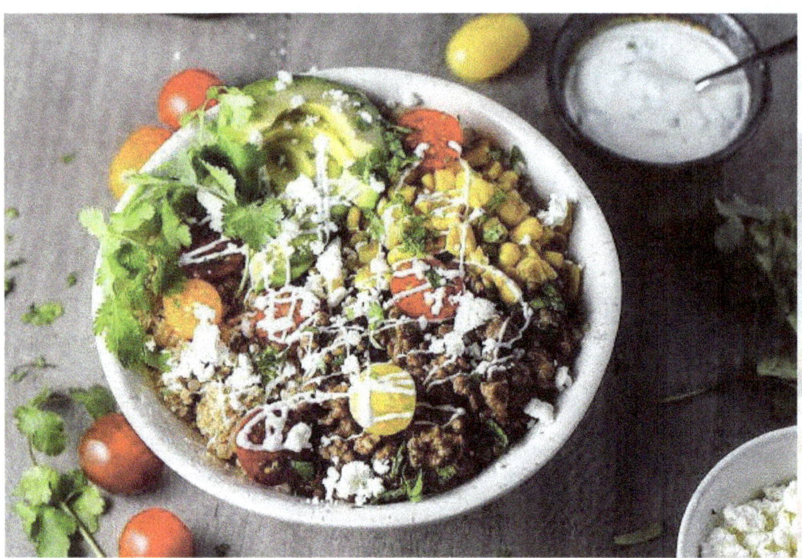

Ingredients:

- 1 cup quinoa, rinsed
- 2 cups water or vegetable broth
- One can (15 oz) of rinsed and drained black beans
- 1 cup corn kernels (fresh or frozen)
- 1 cup cherry tomatoes, halved
- 1 avocado, diced
- 1/2 cup red onion, finely chopped
- 1/4 cup fresh cilantro, chopped
- 1 lime, juiced
- 2 tablespoons olive oil
- 1 teaspoon ground cumin
- 1 teaspoon chili powder
- Salt and pepper to taste
- Optional toppings: salsa, shredded cheese, sour cream

Procedure:

- In a saucepan, combine quinoa and water/broth. Bring to a boil, then reduce heat, cover, and simmer for 15-20 minutes until quinoa is cooked.
- In a large bowl, combine cooked quinoa, black beans, corn, cherry tomatoes, avocado, red onion, and cilantro.

- Mix the lime juice, olive oil, cumin, chilli powder, salt, and pepper in a small bowl.
- Pour the dressing over the quinoa mixture and toss until well combined.
- Adjust seasoning if needed and let it sit for a few minutes to allow flavors to meld.
- Serve in bowls, adding optional toppings as desired.

Time of Preparation:

- Approximately 30 minutes.

Tips and Tricks:

- Cook quinoa with broth for added flavor.
- Customize with your favorite Mexican toppings.
- Adjust lime juice and spices to suit your taste preferences.

Nutritional Value (Per Serving):

- Calories: ~400
- Protein: ~15g
- Carbohydrates: ~55g
- Fat: ~15g
- Fiber: ~10g

Health Benefits:

- Quinoa provides a complete protein source.
- Rich in fiber, vitamins, and minerals from vegetables.
- Healthy fats from avocado contribute to heart health.

Packaging and Storing:

- For up to three days, store in the refrigerator in sealed containers.
- Keep toppings separate for freshness.
- Reheat in the microwave or enjoy cold as a refreshing salad.

Estimated Cost of Preparation:

- Depending on location and ingredient quality, approximately $10-15.

Precautions:

- Ensure quinoa is thoroughly rinsed to remove bitterness.
- Check for allergies or dietary restrictions before adding optional toppings.

Post Caution:

- Refrigerate promptly to prevent bacterial growth.
- Consume within the recommended storage timeframe for optimal freshness.

Lemon Herb Risotto

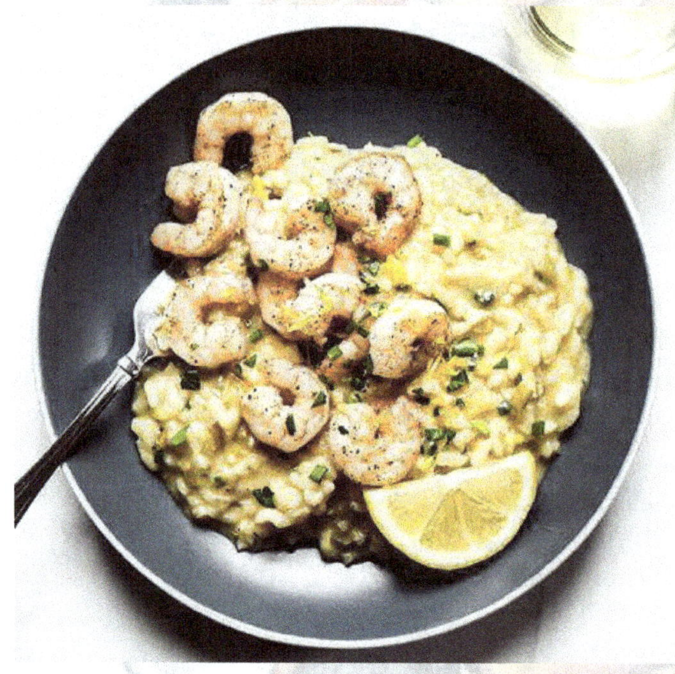

- 1 1/2 cups Arborio rice
- 4 cups vegetable or chicken broth, heated
- 1 cup dry white wine
- 1/2 cup grated Parmesan cheese
- 1/4 cup fresh lemon juice
- Zest of 1 lemon
- 2 tablespoons unsalted butter
- 2 tablespoons olive oil
- 1 small onion, finely chopped
- 2 cloves garlic, minced

- 1/2 cup fresh herbs (parsley, chives, thyme), chopped
- Salt and pepper to taste

- In a large skillet, heat olive oil and 1 tablespoon of butter over medium heat. Add onions and garlic, sauté until softened.
- Add Arborio rice and cook for 2-3 minutes until slightly translucent.
- Add the white wine and whisk until it is mostly absorbed.
- Begin adding heated broth, one ladle at a time, stirring frequently. Don't add extra liquid until the liquid has been mostly absorbed.
- Continue this process until the rice is creamy and al dente, which will take about 18-20 minutes.
- Stir in Parmesan cheese, remaining butter, lemon juice, lemon zest, and chopped herbs. To taste, add salt and pepper for seasoning.
- Before serving, let the risotto sit for a few minutes.

Time of Preparation:

- Approximately 30-35 minutes.

Tips and Tricks:

- Use warm broth to keep the cooking process smooth.
- Constant stirring helps release the rice's starch for creaminess.
- Adjust lemon and herb quantities based on personal preference.

Nutritional Value (Per Serving):

- Calories: ~400
- Protein: ~10g
- Carbohydrates: ~60g
- Fat: ~12g
- Fiber: ~3g

Health Benefits:

- Rich in complex carbohydrates for sustained energy.
- Lemon provides a burst of vitamin C.
- Fresh herbs add antioxidants and flavor without added sodium.

Packaging and Storing:

- Best enjoyed fresh; however, store any leftovers in an airtight container in the refrigerator for up to 2 days.
- Reheat gently on the stovetop with a splash of broth to maintain creaminess.

Estimated Cost of Preparation:

- Depending on location and ingredient quality, approximately $15-20.

Precautions:

- Be attentive during the cooking process to prevent burning.
- Adjust broth quantity if needed; risotto should be creamy, not soupy.

Post Caution:

- Refrigerate promptly to avoid bacterial growth.
- Reheat gently to preserve the creamy texture; add a splash of broth if necessary.

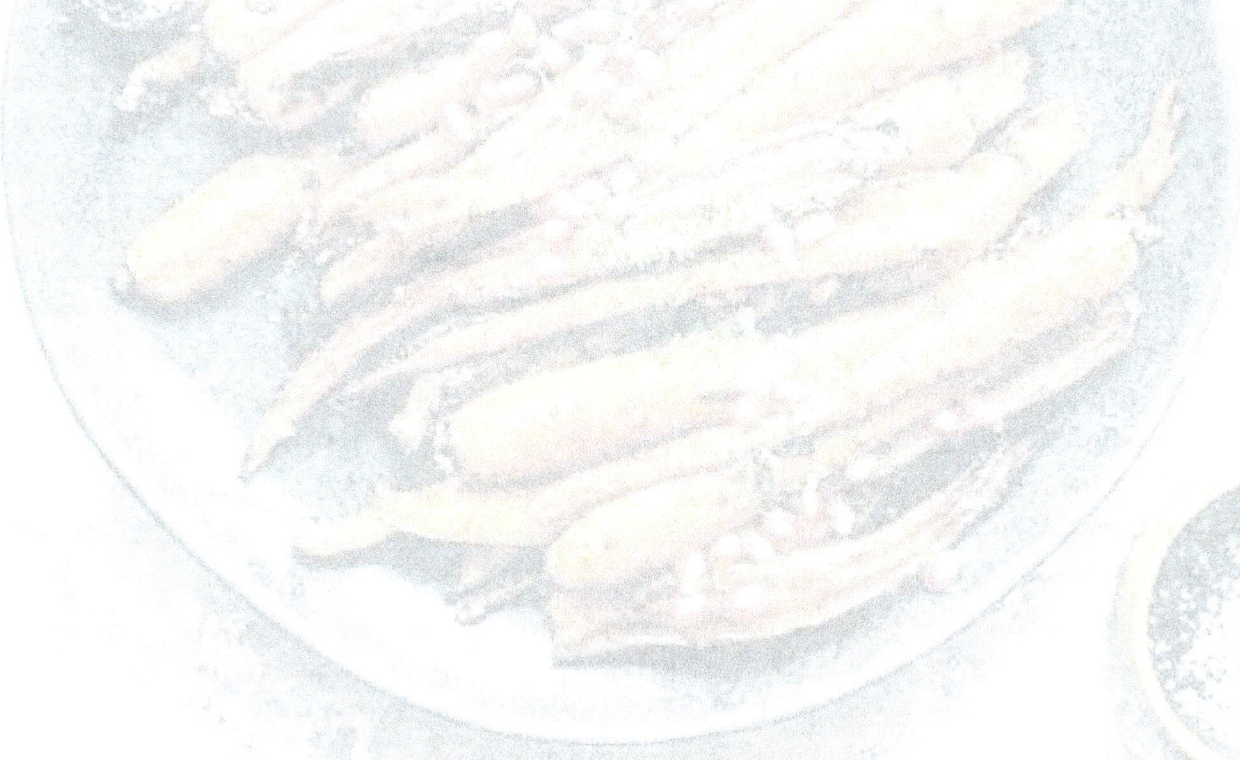

7

Vegetable Side Dishes

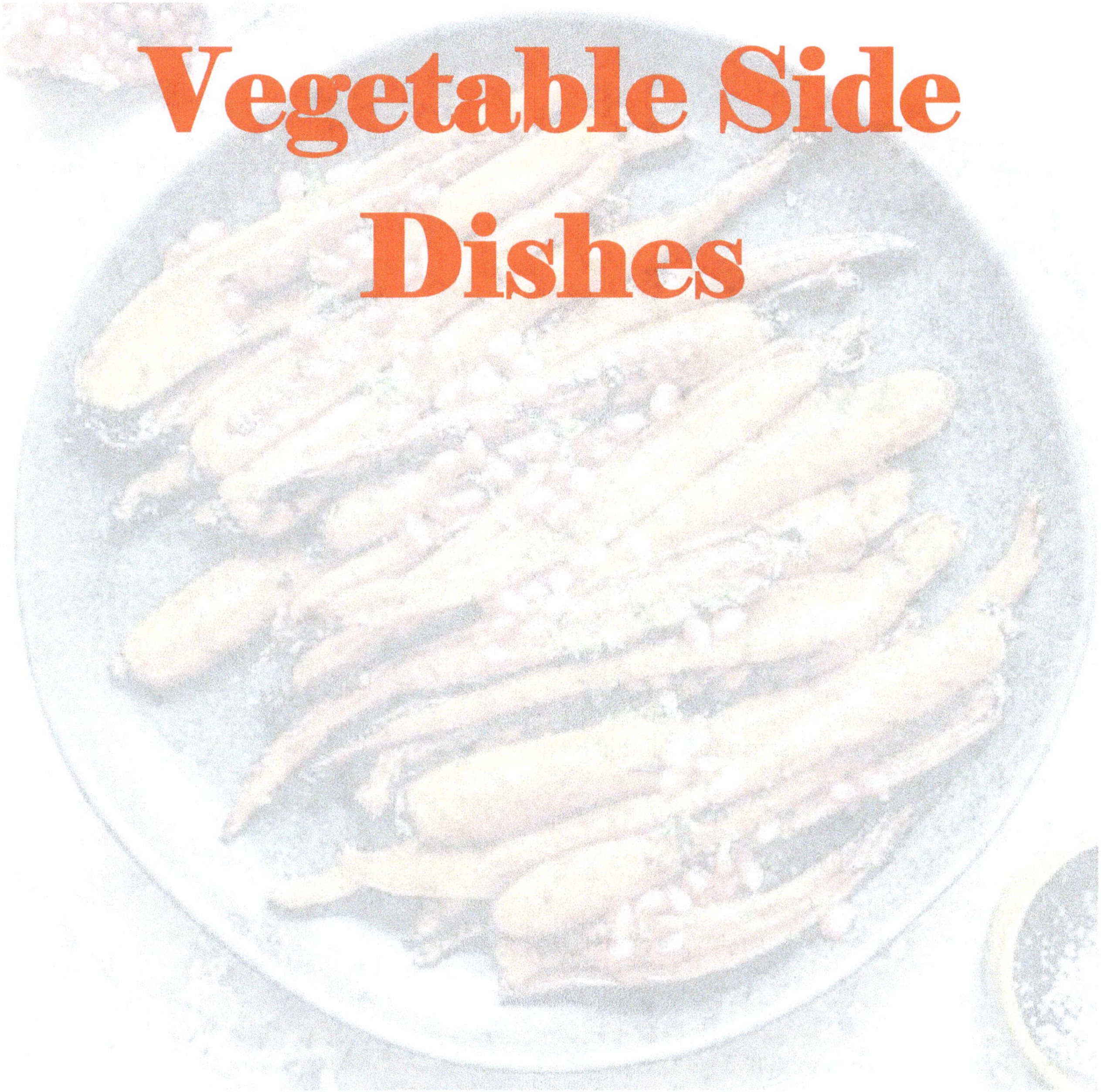

Garlic Parmesan Brussels Sprouts

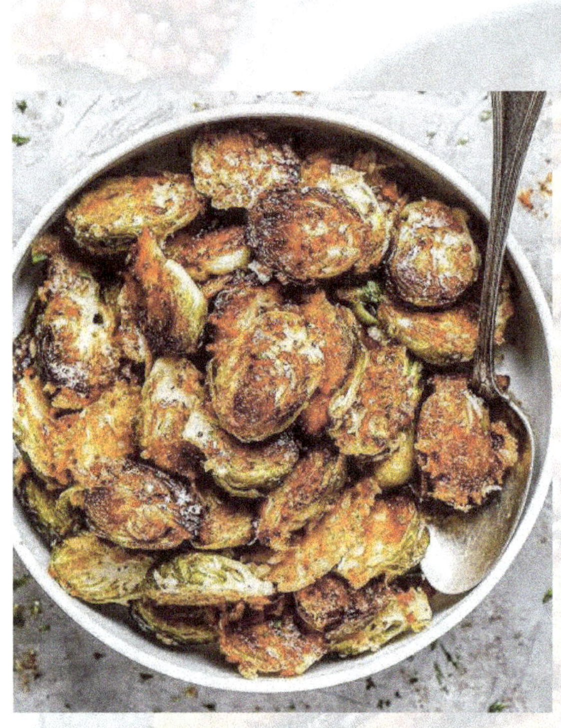

Ingredients:

- 1 lb Brussels sprouts, trimmed and halved
- 3 tbsp olive oil
- 4 cloves garlic, minced
- 1/2 cup grated Parmesan cheese
- Salt and pepper to taste
- 1 tbsp chopped fresh parsley (optional, for garnish)

Procedure:

- Preheat the oven to 400°F (200°C).
- In a large bowl, toss Brussels sprouts with olive oil, minced garlic, salt, and pepper.
- Arrange the Brussels sprouts in a single layer on a baking sheet.
- Roast for 20 to 25 minutes, or until the edges are crispy and golden brown, in a preheated oven.

- Remove from the oven and sprinkle Parmesan cheese over the Brussels sprouts while they are still hot.
- Toss to combine and garnish with chopped parsley if desired.

Time of Preparation:

- Approximately 30 minutes.

Tips and Tricks:

- Ensure Brussels sprouts are evenly coated in oil for crispiness.
- Don't overcrowd the baking sheet to ensure even roasting.
- Adjust salt and pepper to taste.

Nutritional Value (per serving, assuming 4 servings):

- Calories: ~180
- Protein: ~8g
- Fat: ~12g
- Carbohydrates: ~15g
- Fiber: ~6g

Health Benefits:

- Brussels sprouts are high in antioxidants, fibre, and vitamins C and K.
- Garlic has immune-boosting properties.

Packaging and Storing:

- Remaining food can be kept in the refrigerator for up to two days if it is sealed tightly.
- Reheat in the oven for optimal crispiness.

Estimated Cost of Preparation:

- $10-15 (costs may vary based on location and ingredient brands).

Precautions:

- Be cautious when handling hot baking sheets.
- Check for allergies, especially to garlic or Parmesan.

Post-Caution:

- Refrigerate leftovers promptly to avoid spoilage.
- Consume within recommended storage time for the best taste and quality.

Roasted Cauliflower with Tahini Sauce

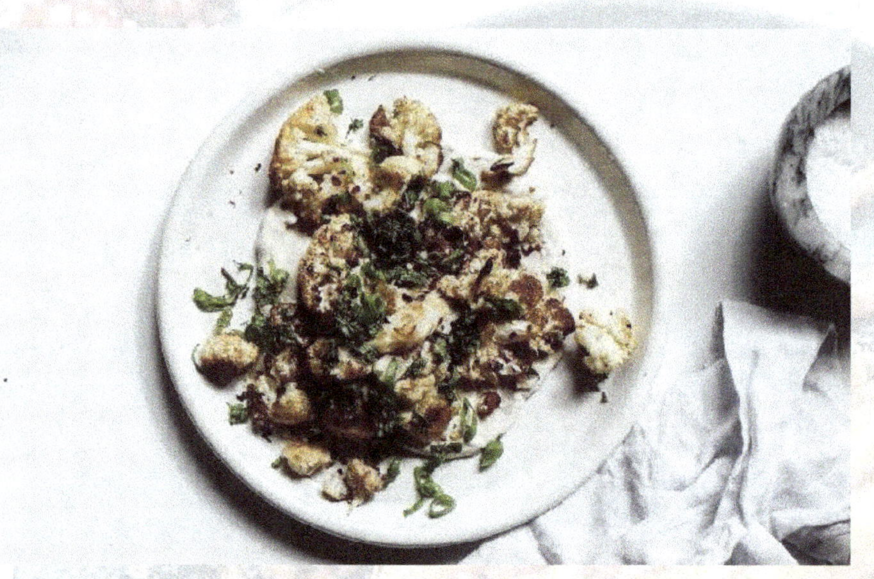

Ingredients:

- 1 large cauliflower, cut into florets
- 3 tbsp olive oil
- 1 tsp ground cumin
- 1 tsp smoked paprika
- Salt and pepper to taste
- 1/2 cup tahini
- 2 tbsp lemon juice
- 2 cloves garlic, minced
- 3-4 tbsp water
- Fresh parsley, chopped (optional, for garnish)

Procedure:

- Preheat the oven to 425°F (220°C).
- In a large bowl, toss cauliflower florets with olive oil, cumin, smoked paprika, salt, and pepper.
- Spread the cauliflower on a baking sheet in a single layer.
- Roast for 25-30 minutes or until golden brown and crisp, tossing halfway through.
- In a small bowl, whisk together tahini, lemon juice, minced garlic, and water until smooth.

- Drizzle the tahini sauce over the roasted cauliflower and garnish with chopped parsley if desired.

Time of Preparation:

- Approximately 40 minutes.

Tips and Tricks:

- Ensure cauliflower florets are evenly coated with seasonings for balanced flavor.
- Adjust tahini sauce consistency with water for desired thickness.
- If you want extra crispiness, broil for a further two to three minutes..

Nutritional Value (per serving, assuming 4 servings):

- Calories: ~220
- Protein: ~7g
- Fat: ~18g
- Carbohydrates: ~10g
- Fiber: ~4g

Health Benefits:

- Cauliflower is rich in vitamins C and K, and fiber.
- Tahini provides healthy fats and is a good source of plant-based protein.

Packaging and Storing:

- Remaining food can be kept in the refrigerator for up to three days if it is sealed tightly.
- Reheat in the oven to maintain crispiness.

Estimated Cost of Preparation:

- $12-18 (costs may vary based on location and ingredient brands).

Precautions:

- Use caution when handling hot baking sheets and roasting pans.
- Be mindful of allergies, especially to tahini or garlic.

Post-Caution:

- Refrigerate leftovers promptly.
- Reheat thoroughly before consumption for the best taste and quality.

Honey Glazed Carrots

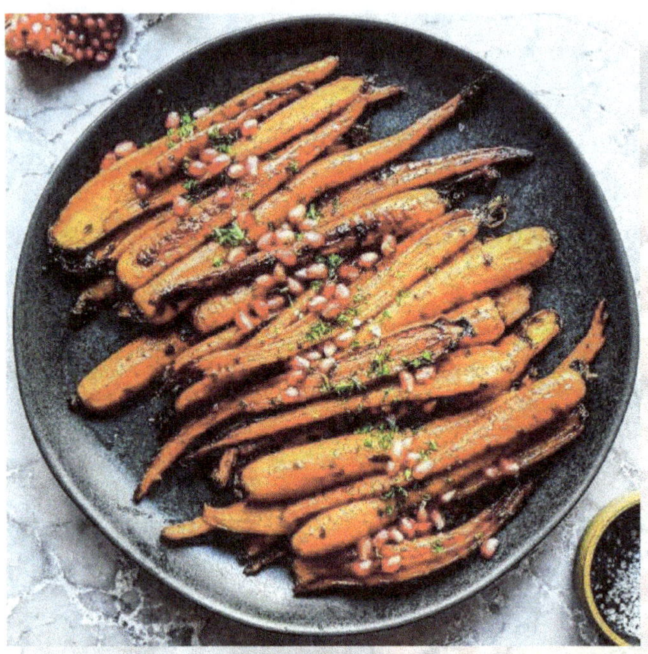

Ingredients:

- 1 lb baby carrots, peeled and trimmed
- 2 tbsp unsalted butter
- 2 tbsp honey
- 1 tbsp fresh parsley, chopped (optional, for garnish)
- Salt and pepper to taste

Procedure:

- Heat the water in a medium-sized saucepan until it boils.
- Add the baby carrots and cook for 5-7 minutes or until they are tender but still have a slight crunch.
- Drain the carrots and set them aside.
- Melt the butter in the same saucepan over a medium heat.
- Add honey to the melted butter, stirring until well combined.
- Add the cooked carrots to the honey-butter mixture, tossing to coat evenly.
- Cook for an additional 2-3 minutes, allowing the carrots to caramelize.
- Season with salt and pepper to taste, garnish with chopped parsley if desired.

Time of Preparation:

- Approximately 20 minutes.

Tips and Tricks:

- Use baby carrots for uniform cooking.
- Adjust honey quantity based on desired sweetness.
- Stir frequently to ensure even glazing.

Nutritional Value (per serving, assuming 4 servings):

- Calories: ~120
- Protein: ~1g
- Fat: ~6g
- Carbohydrates: ~18g
- Fiber: ~3g

Health Benefits:

- Beta-carotene, which is abundant in carrots, is good for the eyes.
- In addition to being naturally sweet, honey contains antioxidants.

Packaging and Storing:

- For up to three days, keep in the refrigerator in an airtight container.
- Reheat in the microwave or on the stovetop.

Estimated Cost of Preparation:

- $8-12 (costs may vary based on location and ingredient brands).

Precautions:

- Be cautious when handling hot saucepans.
- Check for allergies, especially to honey.

Post-Caution:

- Refrigerate leftovers promptly.
- Reheat thoroughly before consumption for the best taste and quality.

8

Protein-Packed Main Courses

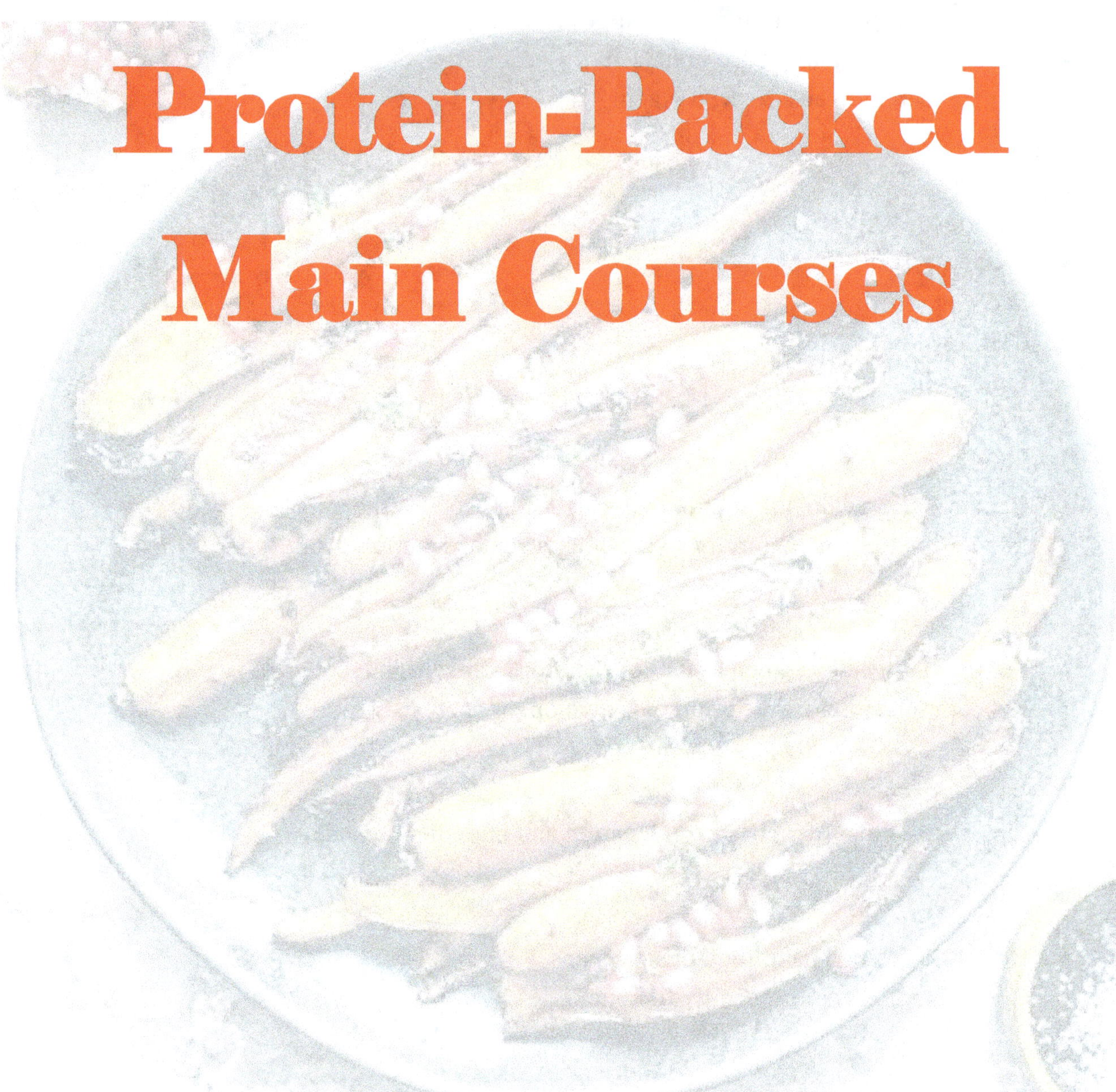

Black Bean and Corn Chili

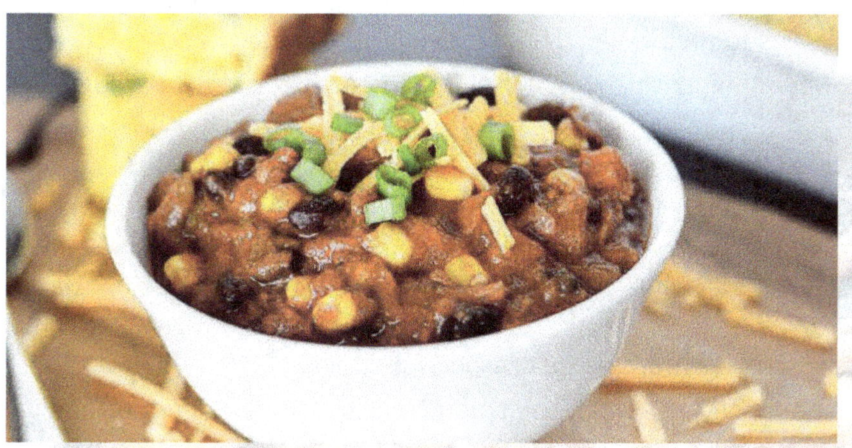

- 1 tablespoon olive oil
- 1 large onion, diced
- 3 cloves garlic, minced
- 1 red bell pepper, diced
- 1 green bell pepper, diced
- One jalapeño jalapeno, cut finely (optional for added heat)
- Two cans (15 ounces each) of rinsed and drained black beans
- 1 can (15 ounces) sweet corn, drained
- 1 can (28 ounces) crushed tomatoes
- 1 cup vegetable broth
- 2 teaspoons ground cumin
- 1 tablespoon chili powder
- 1 teaspoon smoked paprika
- Salt and pepper to taste
- Fresh cilantro, chopped, for garnish
- Lime wedges, for serving

Procedures:

- Warm up the olive oil in a big pot over medium heat. Saute the chopped onions till they become transparent.

- Add minced garlic, diced red and green bell peppers, and jalapeño (if using). Cook until peppers are tender.
- Stir in black beans, sweet corn, crushed tomatoes, and vegetable broth.
- Add ground cumin, chili powder, smoked paprika, salt, and pepper. Mix well.
- After bringing the chilli to a simmer, turn down the heat. Cover and let it cook for about 20-30 minutes, allowing flavors to meld.
- Adjust seasoning to taste. Serve hot, garnished with chopped cilantro and lime wedges.

Time of Preparation:

- Approximately 45 minutes.

Tips and Tricks:

- For a smokier flavor, consider using fire-roasted crushed tomatoes.
- Adjust the chili powder and jalapeño to control the spiciness according to your preference.

Nutritional Value per Serving:

- Calories: Approximately 300 kcal
- Protein: 15g
- Carbohydrates: 55g
- Fat: 5g
- Fiber: 12g

Health Benefits:

- High in fiber, promoting digestive health.
- Rich in plant-based protein.
- Contains antioxidants from various vegetables.

Packaging and Storing:

- Allow the chili to cool before storing in airtight containers.
- For extended storage, freeze or refrigerate for up to 3–4 days.

Estimated Cost of Preparation:

- Cost may vary, but typically ranges from $15 to $20 for a batch serving 4-6 people.

Precautions:

- Be cautious with handling hot peppers; use gloves and avoid touching your face.
- Adjust spice levels according to your tolerance.

- Reheat the chili thoroughly before serving leftovers.
- Consider adding fresh lime or cilantro for a burst of flavor.

Lentil Curry

Ingredients:

- 1 cup dry lentils (green or brown), rinsed and drained
- 1 tablespoon vegetable oil
- 1 large onion, finely chopped
- 3 cloves garlic, minced
- 1 tablespoon ginger, grated
- 1 can (15 ounces) diced tomatoes
- 1 can (15 ounces) coconut milk
- 2 teaspoons curry powder
- 1 teaspoon ground cumin
- 1 teaspoon ground coriander
- 1/2 teaspoon turmeric
- 1/2 teaspoon chili powder (adjust to taste)
- Salt and pepper to taste

- Fresh cilantro, chopped, for garnish
- Cooked rice or naan, for serving

- Vegetable oil should be heated over medium heat in a big pot. Chop the onions and cook them until they get golden brown..
- Add minced garlic and grated ginger. Cook for another minute until fragrant.
- Stir in curry powder, cumin, coriander, turmeric, and chili powder. Toasted the spices by cooking them for a few minutes.
- Add rinsed lentils, diced tomatoes, and coconut milk. Bring to a boil.
- Once the lentils are soft, reduce the heat to low, cover, and simmer for 25 to 30 minutes.
- Season with salt and pepper to taste. Serve over rice or with naan, garnished with chopped cilantro.

Time of Preparation:

- Approximately 45 minutes.

Tips and Tricks:

- Use red lentils for a quicker cooking time.
- Experiment with different curry powders for varied flavor profiles.

Nutritional Value per Serving:

- Calories: Approximately 350 kcal
- Protein: 15g
- Carbohydrates: 45g
- Fat: 15g
- Fiber: 12g

Health Benefits:

- High in plant-based protein and fiber.
- Rich in essential vitamins and minerals.
- Coconut milk adds healthy fats.

Packaging and Storing:

- Allow the curry to cool before storing in airtight containers.
- For extended storage, freeze or refrigerate for up to 3–4 days.

- Cost may vary, but typically ranges from $10 to $15 for a batch serving 4-6 people.

Precautions:

- Check lentils for debris before cooking.
- Adjust chili powder to control spiciness.

Post-Caution:

- Reheat thoroughly before serving leftovers.
- Consider adding a splash of coconut milk or a squeeze of lime for added freshness.

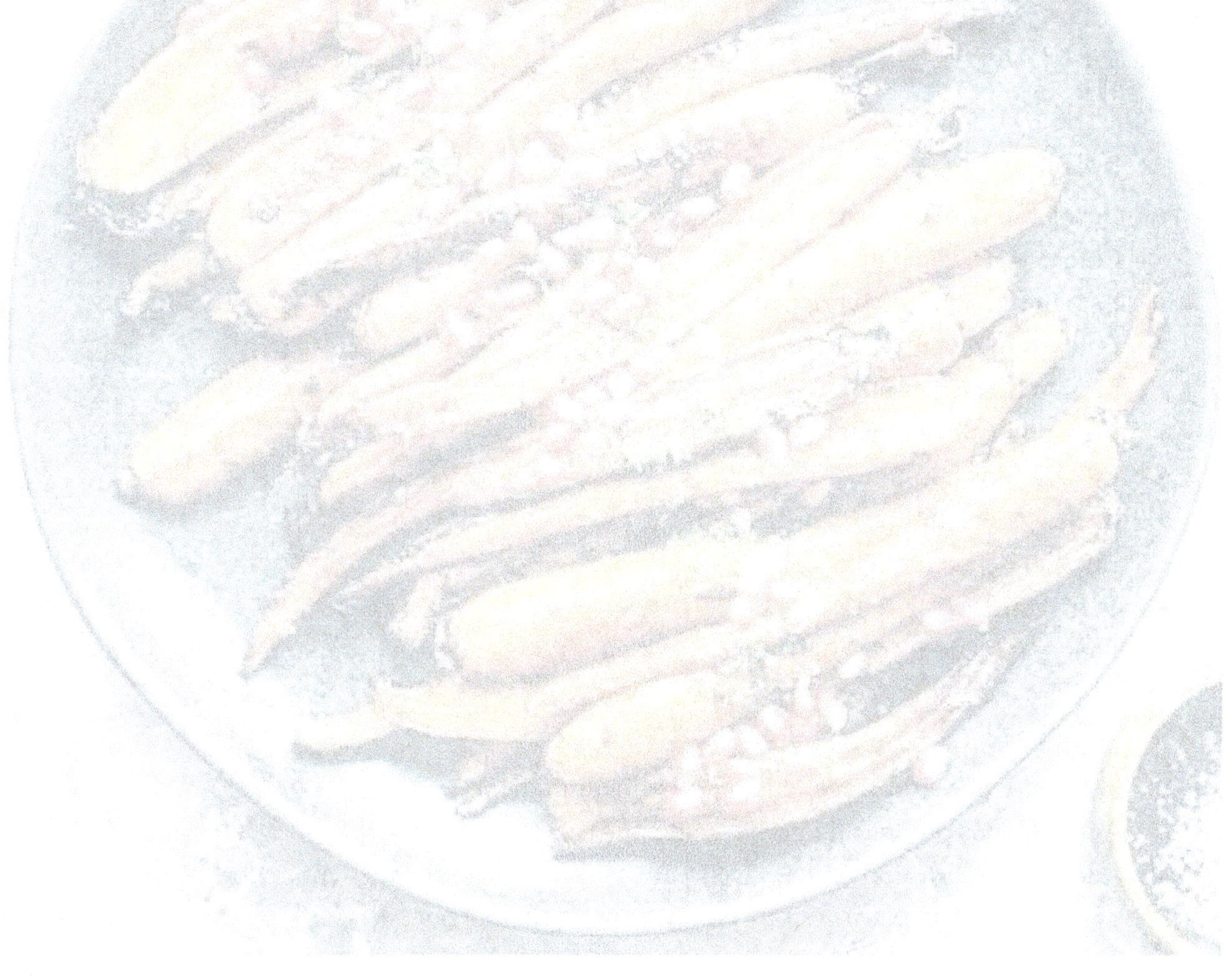

BBQ Jackfruit Tacos

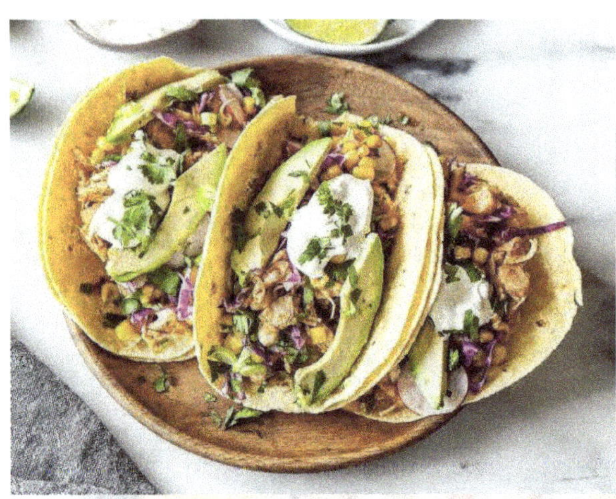

Ingredients:

- 2 cans (20 ounces each) young green jackfruit in water, drained and rinsed
- 1 tablespoon vegetable oil
- 1 small onion, finely chopped
- 2 cloves garlic, minced
- 1/2 cup barbecue sauce
- 1 teaspoon smoked paprika
- 1/2 teaspoon cumin
- 1/2 teaspoon chili powder
- Salt and pepper to taste
- Corn tortillas
- Toppings: Shredded cabbage, diced tomatoes, avocado slices, cilantro, lime wedges

Procedures:

- In a skillet, heat the vegetable oil over medium heat.
- Add chopped onions and garlic, sauté until softened.
- Add jackfruit to the skillet. As it cooks, shred the jackfruit with a fork.Stir in barbecue sauce, smoked paprika, cumin, chili powder, salt, and pepper. Cook for 10-15 minutes until jackfruit absorbs the flavors.
- Warm corn tortillas. Spoon the BBQ jackfruit onto each tortilla.
- Top with shredded cabbage, diced tomatoes, avocado slices, cilantro, and a squeeze of lime.

Time of Preparation:

- Approximately 30 minutes.

Tips and Tricks:

- Choose young green jackfruit in water, not in syrup, for savory dishes.
- Adjust barbecue sauce and spices to your taste preferences.

Nutritional Value per Serving:

- Calories: Approximately 200 kcal
- Protein: 2g
- Carbohydrates: 40g
- Fat: 5g
- Fiber: 5g

Health Benefits:

- Jackfruit is a good source of dietary fiber.
- Low in calories and fat compared to traditional meat-based tacos.

Packaging and Storing:

- Allow the BBQ jackfruit to cool before storing in airtight containers.
- Refrigerate for up to 3-4 days.

Estimated Cost of Preparation:

- Cost may vary, but typically ranges from $12 to $18 for a batch serving 4-6 people.

Precautions:

- Check jackfruit for seeds and remove them before cooking.
- Adjust spice levels according to your preference.

Post-Caution:

- Reheat thoroughly before serving leftovers.
- Freshen up tacos with additional toppings like salsa or guacamole.

Chocolate Lava Cake

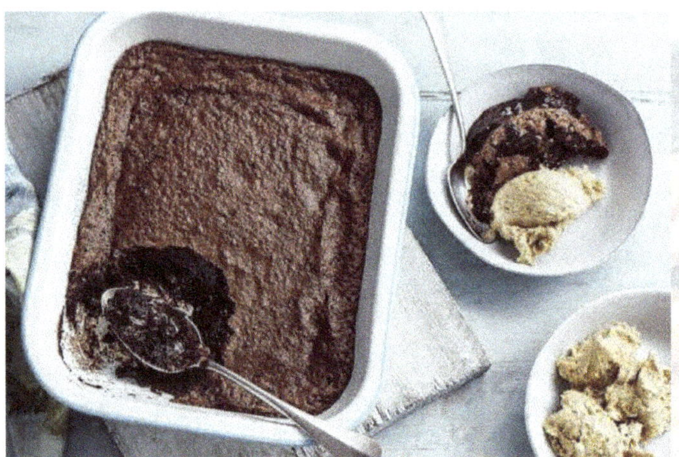

Ingredients:

- 1/2 cup unsalted butter
- 1 cup semi-sweet chocolate chips
- 1/2 cup powdered sugar
- 2 large eggs
- 2 large egg yolks
- 1 teaspoon vanilla extract
- 1/4 cup all-purpose flour
- Pinch of salt
- Cocoa powder for dusting (optional)
- Whipping cream or vanilla ice cream to serve

Procedures:

- Preheat the oven to 425°F (220°C). Grease and flour individual ramekins.
- In a microwave-safe bowl, melt the butter and chocolate chips in 30-second intervals until smooth.
- Stir in powdered sugar until well combined.
- In a separate bowl, whisk together eggs, egg yolks, and vanilla extract. Add this to the chocolate mixture and mix well.
- Fold in flour and salt after sifting until just incorporated. Avoid over-mixing.
- After the ramekins are ready, evenly divide the batter among them.
- Bake for 12-14 minutes or until the edges are set, but the center is still soft.

- Allow the cakes to cool for a minute, then run a knife around the edges and invert onto serving plates.
- Dust with cocoa powder and serve immediately with vanilla ice cream or whipped cream.

Time of Preparation:

- Approximately 20 minutes.

Tips and Tricks:

- Ensure the ramekins are well-greased and floured for easy release.
- Be cautious not to overbake; the center should be gooey for the lava effect.

Nutritional Value per Serving:

- Calories: Approximately 400 kcal
- Protein: 5g
- Carbohydrates: 35g
- Fat: 28g
- Sugar: 28g

Health Benefits:

- Indulgent treat; consume in moderation.
- Dark chocolate may provide antioxidants and improve mood.

Packaging and Storing:

- Best served fresh; however, you can refrigerate any leftovers and reheat for a short time in the microwave.

Estimated Cost of Preparation:

- Cost may vary, but typically ranges from $10 to $15 for a batch serving 4-6 people.

Precautions:

- Be cautious handling hot ramekins; use oven mitts.
- Monitor baking time to achieve the desired lava consistency.

Post-Caution:

- Enjoy immediately for the best lava experience.
- Consider adding a scoop of vanilla ice cream for extra decadence.
- Indulge in the rich and gooey delight of Chocolate Lava Cake!

Rice Pudding

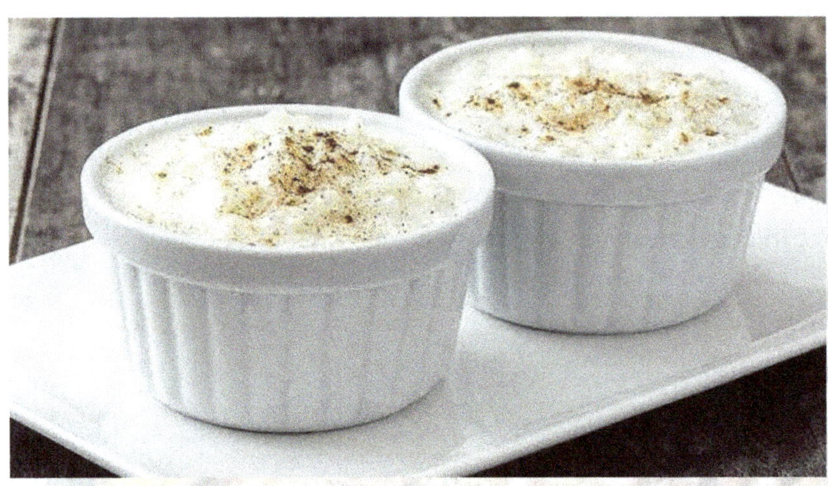

- 1 cup white rice
- 4 cups whole milk
- 1/2 cup granulated sugar
- 1/2 teaspoon vanilla extract
- 1/4 teaspoon ground cinnamon
- Pinch of salt
- Raisins or nutmeg for garnish (optional)

Procedures:

- Till the water runs clear, rinse the rice under cold water.
- In a medium-sized saucepan, combine the rinsed rice, whole milk, sugar, vanilla extract, ground cinnamon, and a pinch of salt.
- Bring the mixture to a boil over medium-high heat, then reduce the heat to low and simmer, stirring frequently.
- Cook for 25-30 minutes or until the rice is tender and the mixture has thickened to a creamy consistency.
- Remove from heat and let it stand for a few minutes. If desired, stir in raisins or sprinkle with nutmeg for extra flavor.
- Serve warm or chilled. Refrigerate any leftovers.

- Approximately 40 minutes.

- Stir the rice pudding frequently to prevent it from sticking to the bottom of the pan.
- Adjust sugar and cinnamon to taste preferences.

- Calories: Approximately 200 kcal
- Protein: 5g
- Carbohydrates: 35g
- Fat: 5g
- Calcium: 15% DV

- Good source of calcium from whole milk.
- Provides energy from carbohydrates.
- Comforting and easy-to-digest dessert.

- Allow the rice pudding to cool before storing in airtight containers.
- Refrigerate for up to 3-4 days.

- Cost may vary, but typically ranges from $5 to $10 for a batch serving 4-6 people.

- Be cautious when cooking to avoid scalding from hot milk.
- To keep the rice from sticking, stir it often.

- Reheat gently in a saucepan with a splash of milk if the pudding thickens too much.
- Enjoy the rice pudding as is or with a sprinkle of cinnamon.

Berry Compote

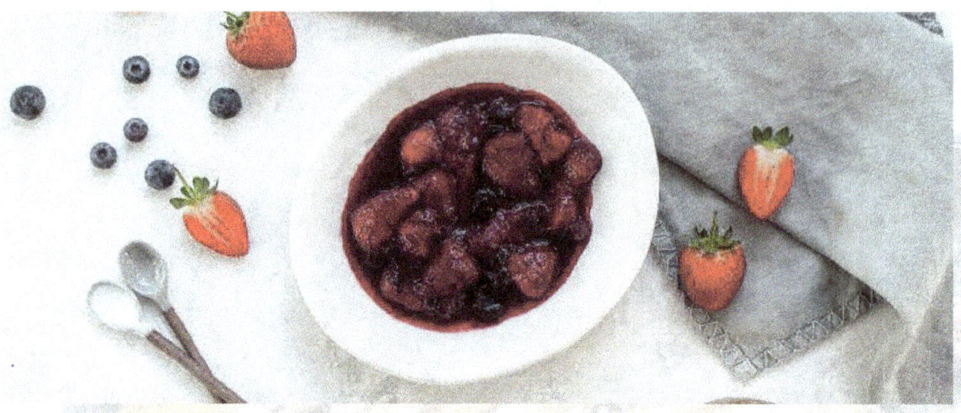

- Two cups of mixed berries, including blackberries, raspberries, blueberries, and strawberries
- 1/4 cup granulated sugar
- 1 tablespoon lemon juice
- 1 teaspoon cornstarch (optional, for thickening)
- 1/2 teaspoon vanilla extract (optional)

Procedures:

- Wash and prepare the berries as needed. If using strawberries, hull and slice them.
- In a saucepan, combine the mixed berries, granulated sugar, and lemon juice.
- Heat the mixture over medium heat, stirring gently until the sugar dissolves and the berries release their juices.
- Bring the mixture to a simmer and cook for 8-10 minutes, stirring occasionally, until the berries break down and the compote thickens.
- If desired, mix cornstarch with a little water to create a slurry, then add it to the compote to thicken.
- Take off the heat and, if using, whisk in the vanilla essence..
- Let the compote cool slightly before serving. It will continue to thicken as it cools.

Time of Preparation:

- Approximately 15 minutes.

- Use a mix of berries for a flavorful combination.
- Adjust sugar to taste depending on the sweetness of the berries.

Nutritional Value per Serving:

- Calories: Approximately 50 kcal
- Carbohydrates: 12g
- Fiber: 3g
- Vitamin C: 15% DV

Health Benefits:

- High in antioxidants and vitamins from the berries.
- Low in calories and a delicious topping for various dishes.

Packaging and Storing:

- Allow the berry compote to cool before transferring it to airtight containers.
- For extended storage, freeze or refrigerate for up to one week.

Estimated Cost of Preparation:

- Cost may vary, but typically ranges from $5 to $8 for a batch serving 4-6 people.

Precautions:

- Be cautious when simmering to avoid splattering.
- Adjust sweetness based on personal preference.

Post-Caution:

- Serve the berry compote over pancakes, waffles, yogurt, or ice cream.
- Experiment with different berries for unique flavor profiles.

9

Special Occasion Dishes

Stuffed Bell Peppers

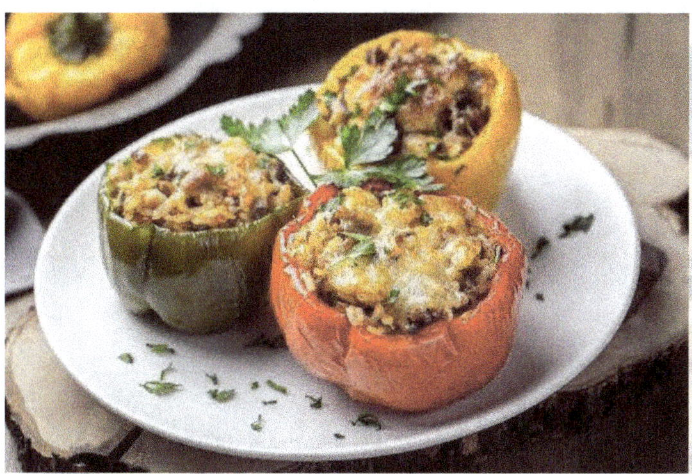

Ingredients:

- 4 large bell peppers (any color)
- 1 lb ground beef or turkey
- 1 cup cooked rice
- 1 cup black beans, drained and rinsed
- 1 cup corn kernels
- 1 cup diced tomatoes
- 1 cup shredded cheese (cheddar or your preference)
- 1/2 cup diced onion
- 2 cloves garlic, minced
- 1 teaspoon cumin
- 1 teaspoon chili powder
- Salt and pepper to taste
- 1 cup tomato sauce

Procedures:

- Preheat the oven to 375°F (190°C).
- Remove the seeds and membranes from the bell peppers by cutting off the tops.
- Cook the ground meat until browned in a pan.
- . Drain excess fat.
- In a large bowl, mix cooked meat, rice, black beans, corn, tomatoes, cheese, onion, garlic, cumin, chili powder, salt, and pepper.

- Stuff each bell pepper with the mixture.
- Pour tomato sauce into a baking dish, place stuffed peppers, and cover with foil.
- Bake peppers for 25 to 30 minutes, or until soft.
- Remove foil, sprinkle extra cheese on top, and bake uncovered for an additional 10 minutes.

Time of Preparation:

- Approximately 45-50 minutes.

Tips and Tricks:

- Use a variety of bell pepper colors for a visually appealing dish.
- Pre-cook bell peppers in boiling water for 5 minutes if you prefer a softer texture.
- Experiment with different cheeses for added flavor.

Nutritional Value (per serving):

- Calories: ~400
- Protein: ~20g
- Carbohydrates: ~40g
- Fat: ~18g
- Fiber: ~8g

Health Benefits:

- Rich in protein and fiber.
- High in vitamins A and C from bell peppers.

Packaging and Storing:

- Remaining food can be kept in the refrigerator for up to three days if it is sealed tightly.

Estimated Cost of Preparation:

- Depending on local prices, approximately $15-$20 for 4 servings.

Precautions:

- Ensure ground meat is thoroughly cooked.
- Be cautious while handling hot peppers.

Post-Caution:

- Refrigerate leftovers promptly to prevent spoilage.

- Reheat thoroughly before consuming.

Eggplant Parmesan

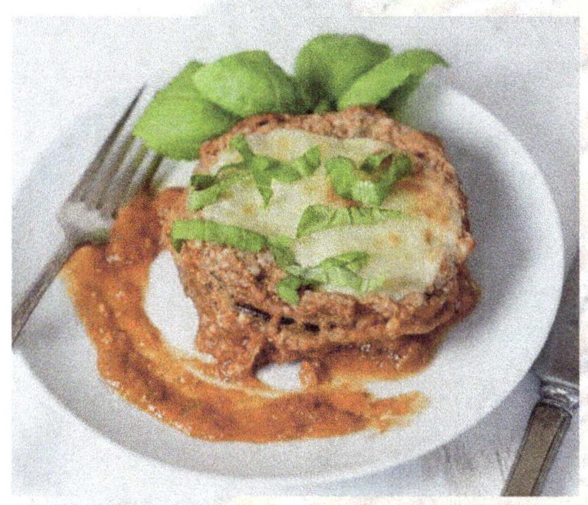

- 2 large eggplants, sliced into 1/2-inch rounds
- 2 cups breadcrumbs
- 1 cup grated Parmesan cheese
- 4 cups marinara sauce
- 2 cups shredded mozzarella cheese
- 1 cup all-purpose flour
- 4 large eggs, beaten
- 2 teaspoons dried oregano
- 2 teaspoons dried basil
- Salt and pepper to taste
- Fresh basil for garnish (optional)

Procedures:

- Preheat the oven to 375°F (190°C).

- Sprinkle eggplant slices with salt, let them sit for 30 minutes, then pat dry to remove excess moisture.
- Set up a breading station with flour, beaten eggs, and a mixture of breadcrumbs, Parmesan, oregano, basil, salt, and pepper.
- Dredge eggplant slices in flour, dip in eggs, and coat with breadcrumb mixture.
- Heat oil in a skillet and fry eggplant slices until golden brown. Drain excess oil on paper towels.
- In a baking dish, spread a thin layer of marinara sauce, place a layer of fried eggplant, and sprinkle with mozzarella. Repeat layers.
- Finish with a layer of marinara and mozzarella on top.
- Bake for 25 to 30 minutes, or until brown and bubbling.
- Garnish with fresh basil if desired.

Time of Preparation:

- Approximately 1 hour.

Tips and Tricks:

- Use panko breadcrumbs for extra crispiness.
- Bake on a rack for a crisper bottom layer.
- To ensure uniform cooking, make sure to slice the aubergine evenly.

Nutritional Value (per serving):

- Calories: ~350
- Protein: ~15g
- Carbohydrates: ~35g
- Fat: ~15g
- Fiber: ~8g

Health Benefits:

- Good source of dietary fiber.
- Provides vitamins and minerals, including potassium and vitamin C.

Packaging and Storing:

- Remaining food can be kept in the refrigerator for up to three days if it is sealed tightly.

Estimated Cost of Preparation:

- Depending on local prices, approximately $12-$15 for 4 servings.

Precautions:

- Be careful when frying eggplant slices to avoid oil splatter.
- Watch out for hot surfaces when assembling layers.

Post-Caution:

- Allow the dish to cool before serving.
- Refrigerate leftovers promptly to prevent spoilage.

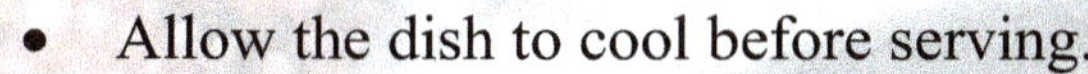

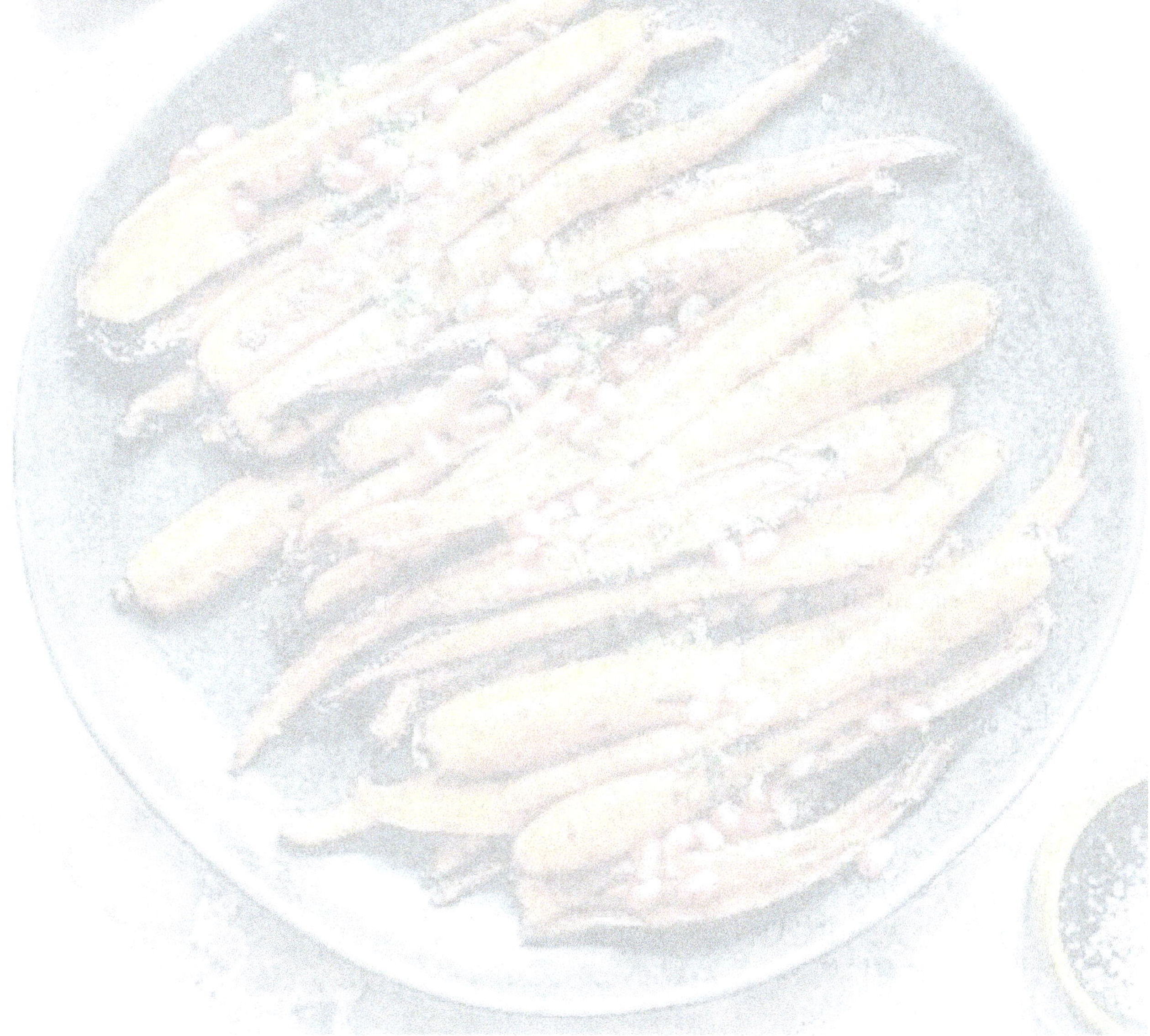

Quinoa-Stuffed Acorn Squash

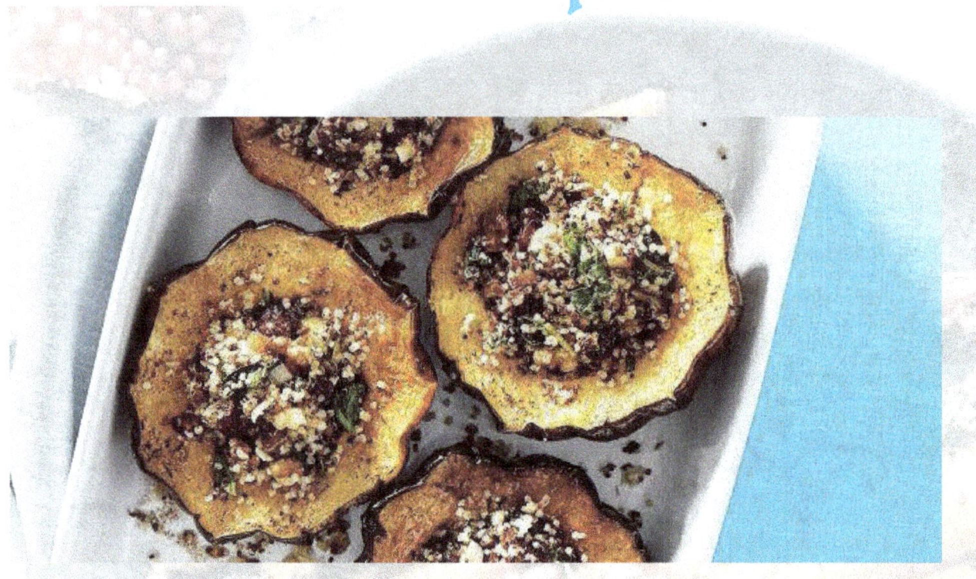

Ingredients:

- 2 acorn squash, halved and seeds removed
- 1 cup quinoa, rinsed
- 2 cups vegetable broth
- 1 cup chickpeas, cooked
- 1 cup diced apples
- 1/2 cup dried cranberries
- 1/2 cup chopped pecans
- 1/4 cup chopped fresh parsley
- 2 tablespoons olive oil
- 1 teaspoon ground cinnamon
- 1/2 teaspoon ground cumin
- Salt and pepper to taste

Procedures:

- Preheat the oven to 400°F (200°C).
- Brush the inside of acorn squash halves with olive oil and sprinkle with salt and pepper.
- Place squash halves on a baking sheet and bake for 25-30 minutes or until tender.

- In a saucepan, combine quinoa and vegetable broth. Bring to a boil, then reduce heat, cover, and simmer for 15-20 minutes until quinoa is cooked.
- In a large bowl, mix cooked quinoa, chickpeas, apples, cranberries, pecans, parsley, olive oil, cinnamon, cumin, salt, and pepper.
- After roasting, spoon the quinoa mixture into the halves of acorn squash.
- Bake for an additional 15 minutes until heated through.

Time of Preparation:

- Approximately 1 hour.

Tips and Tricks:

- Choose small acorn squash for a better balance between squash and stuffing.
- Toast pecans for added flavor and crunch.

Nutritional Value (per serving):

- Calories: ~400
- Protein: ~10g
- Carbohydrates: ~60g
- Fat: ~15g
- Fiber: ~10g
- Health Benefits:
- High in fiber and protein.
- Rich in vitamins A and C from acorn squash.

Packaging and Storing:

- Remaining food can be kept in the refrigerator for up to three days if it is sealed tightly.

Estimated Cost of Preparation:

- Depending on local prices, approximately $10-$15 for 4 servings.

Precautions:

- Be cautious when handling hot squash.

Post-Caution:

- Allow the dish to cool before serving.
- Refrigerate leftovers promptly to prevent spoilage.

10

Healthy Instant Pot Hacks

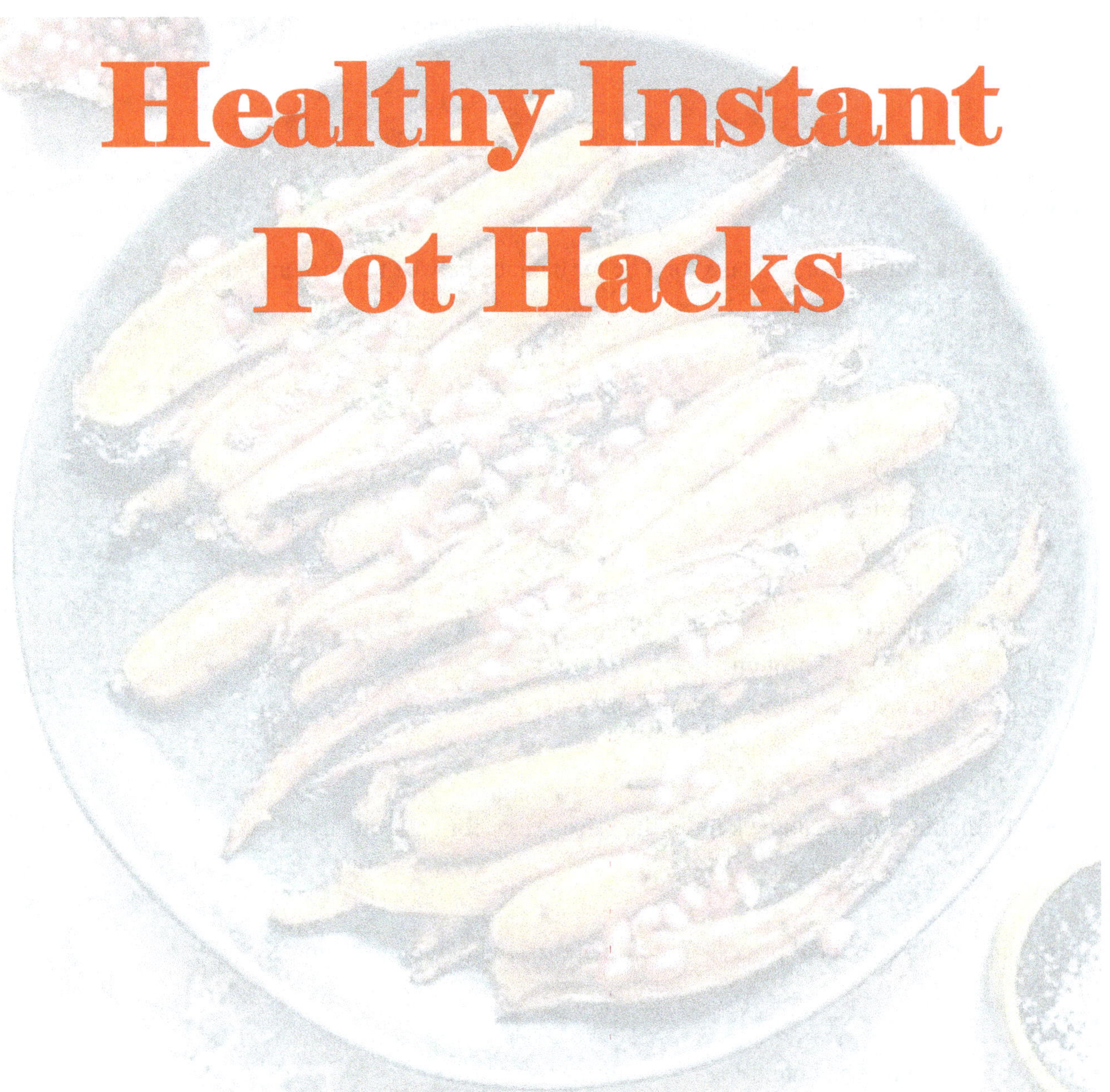

Substitutions For Healthier Options

- Whole Grains Instead of White Rice: Opt for brown rice, quinoa, or farro for a higher fiber content and additional nutrients.
- Lean Proteins: Choose lean meats like chicken breast, turkey, or lean cuts of pork instead of fattier options to reduce saturated fat intake.
- Vegetable Broth Instead of Oil: Saute vegetables using vegetable broth instead of oil to cut down on unnecessary calories and saturated fats.
- Greek Yogurt Instead of Sour Cream: Swap sour cream with Greek yogurt for a creamy texture with added protein and probiotics.
- Cauliflower Rice as a Low-Carb Alternative: Replace traditional rice with cauliflower rice to reduce carbohydrates and increase vegetable intake.
- Homemade Spice Blends Instead of Pre-Packaged Seasonings:
- Create your spice blends to control sodium levels and avoid unnecessary additives in pre-packaged seasonings.
- Natural Sweeteners: Opt for natural sweeteners like honey or maple syrup instead of refined sugar for a healthier sweetness.
- Low-Sodium Broth: Choose low-sodium broth to control your salt intake while still adding flavor to your dishes.
- Steam Vegetables Instead of Boiling: Use the Instant Pot's steaming function to cook vegetables quickly, preserving more nutrients compared to boiling.
- Beans Instead of Meat: Incorporate beans or lentils as a protein source in place of meat for a plant-based alternative.
- Homemade Tomato Sauce: Make your own tomato sauce using fresh tomatoes and herbs to avoid added sugars and preservatives found in store-bought versions.
- Add Greens at the End: Stir in leafy greens like spinach or kale at the end of the cooking process to retain their nutritional value.
- Use the Trivet for Cooking Protein and Veggies Together:
- Utilize the trivet to cook proteins and vegetables simultaneously, saving time and energy.
- Portion Control: Be mindful of portion sizes to avoid overeating, even with healthier ingredients.

- Experiment with Herbs and Spices: Enhance flavors with a variety of herbs and spices, reducing the need for excessive salt or unhealthy condiments.

By incorporating these substitutions and hacks, you can transform your Instant Pot recipes into healthier, nutrient-packed meals without sacrificing flavor.

Cooking Tips For Maximizing Nutrients

- Use Minimal Water: When cooking in the Instant Pot, use just enough water or broth to cover the ingredients. This helps retain more water-soluble vitamins and minerals.
- Quick Cooking for Vegetables: Opt for the "Zero Minutes" setting or very short cooking times for vegetables to prevent nutrient loss. The residual heat will continue cooking them without overdoing it.
- Preserve Phytonutrients with Quick Release: For ingredients rich in phytonutrients (such as colorful vegetables), use the quick release method to preserve their vibrant colors and nutritional content.
- Prefer Steaming Over Boiling: Steam vegetables instead of boiling them. Steaming helps retain more nutrients that can leach into the water during boiling.
- Cook Beans and Legumes from Scratch: Prepare beans and legumes in the Instant Pot without pre-soaking to retain more nutrients. The pressure cooking process preserves their nutritional value.
- Add Nutrient-Dense Broths: Use homemade broths made from nutrient-dense ingredients like bones, vegetables, and herbs to infuse your dishes with additional vitamins and minerals.
- Include a Variety of Colors: Incorporate a colorful array of fruits and vegetables in your Instant Pot recipes to ensure a diverse range of nutrients.

- Don't Peel Everything: Keep the skins on fruits and vegetables whenever possible to maximize fiber content and retain nutrients found in or near the skin.
- Utilize Herbs and Spices: Enhance flavors with herbs and spices instead of excessive salt or unhealthy condiments. Many herbs and spices also offer health benefits.
- Choose Whole Grains: Opt for whole grains like brown rice, quinoa, or barley over refined grains to ensure you get the maximum nutritional benefit.
- Add Leafy Greens at the End: Stir in leafy greens such as spinach or kale at the end of the cooking process to preserve their vibrant color and nutritional content.
- Infuse Flavors with Citrus: Add citrus zest or juice at the end of cooking to impart fresh flavors and boost vitamin C content.
- Consider Nutrient Timing: Add ingredients with shorter cooking times towards the end to prevent overcooking and preserve their nutritional value.
- Incorporate Superfoods: Include superfoods like chia seeds, flaxseeds, or hemp seeds at the end of cooking or as a topping to boost omega-3 fatty acids and other essential nutrients.
- Balance Macronutrients: Aim for a well-balanced meal by including a mix of lean proteins, healthy fats, and complex carbohydrates in your Instant Pot recipes.

By applying these cooking tips and Instant Pot hacks, you can optimize the nutritional content of your meals, making them both delicious and health-enhancing.

CONCLUSION

In conclusion, the Instant Pot Vegetarian Recipes Cookbook offers a delightful journey into the world of flavorful and nourishing plant-based meals. With its diverse array of innovative recipes and time-saving techniques, this cookbook not only caters to the culinary needs of vegetarians but also provides a culinary adventure for anyone seeking vibrant, delicious, and hassle-free cooking. Elevate your dining experience with the wholesome and tempting dishes found within these pages, making every meal a celebration of taste and health. Happy cooking!